Diabetes
Home Exercise Guide & Workbook

Plus

Exercise Benefits & Precautions

Lost Temple Fitness & Rehab

Karen Cutler: LPTA, ACE Certified Personal Trainer,
Medical, Cancer, Arthritis & Therapeutic Exercise Specialist

It is advised that you always check with your medical doctor or physical therapist before starting an exercise program or change in diet.

Websites

LostTempleFitness.com

LostTempleNutrition.com

LostTemplePets.com

LostTempleArt.com

LostTempleFitnessCancer.com

Introduction

It has been proven that exercise and nutrition are two of the main factors that you can control for a healthy lifestyle. Many people do not know how to start or progress an exercise program. There are hundreds of pictures for beginner, intermediate and advanced exercise programs, as well as a list of equipment that you can use in the home. This also includes worksheets to help you track your exercises and progress.

The diabetes section includes information on Type 1, 2 and gestational diabetes. This also includes medications and other related issues such as neuropathy and foot issues. Diet and Fitness are a major part of controlling your diabetes, but you also need to know the warning signs of things like hypoglycemia, Ketoacidosis and hyperosmolar hyperglycemic state for a safe exercise routine.

"Diabetes is a disease that occurs when your blood glucose, also called blood sugar, is too high. Over time, having too much glucose in your blood can cause health problems, such as heart disease, nerve damage, eye problems, and kidney disease. You can take steps to prevent diabetes or manage it. An estimated 30.3 million people in the United States, or 9.4 percent of the population, have diabetes. About one in four people with diabetes don't know they have the disease. An estimated 84.1 million Americans aged 18 years or older have prediabetes". (*NIH – National Institute of Diabetes and Digestive and Kidney Diseases (2022).*

This book is for:

- Those with a diagnosis of diabetes, pre-diabetes, neuropathy or metabolic disorders.
- The beginner who has never exercised before
- The individual that has mastered the basics but wants to know how to advance to the next level.
- Pre/post rehab individuals who would like to advance or want a list of exercise programs to follow.
- The personal trainer, physical therapist, or other coaches who would like their client to have a list of exercises that can be progressed.

This book is not for or may need modification:

- Chronic or acute disorders/injury's that is not being followed by a health care professional. This book can be used in conjunction with a rehab program.
- If you are over 40 and have never exercised before, it is advised that a physician clears you first.
- Undiagnosed pain
- The person that does not feel they can safely modify their individual program, although can be used in conjunction with rehab or coaches/personal trainers.
- People with the following issues that have been cleared by an MD for an exercise program or in conjunction with rehab. These issues may be addressed in future volumes: Cardiac disease, Cancer, Respiratory disease and Arthritis.

What is covered in this book?

- Diabetes
    - Type 1, 2 and Gestational Diabetes
    - Diabetic Neuropathy
    - Medications, Insulin & Other Treatments
    - Diabetic Foot Issues
    - Hypoglycemia
    - Physical Activity
    - Diet

- Home Exercise Programs – pictures with explanations and worksheets
    - Myofascial release
    - Flexibility – Stretching
    - Core Stability
    - Balance with progression to Standing Strengthening exercises
    - Strengthening
        - Lower extremity - Lying and Seated
        - Upper extremity
- Benefits and Factors to consider before starting an exercise program
- Vital signs and how to monitor exercise intensity
- Temperature – Heat and Cold
- Dehydration
- Anatomy
- Equipment needed for home exercise
- Self-Tests
- Warm up/cool down
- Duration, Frequency, Intensity and Primary Movement Patterns

It is advised that you always check with your medical doctor or physical therapist beforestarting an exercise program or change in diet.

Disclaimer: The information in this book is for educational purposes only and has been obtained through research, publications and personal experience, and shall not be liable for incorrect information. Any mentioned publications or websites does not imply endorsement. As this industry is ever changing, I urge readers to confirm the information contained in this book.The author will not be liable for any injuries sustained from practicing techniques taught in this book or for any typographical errors or omissions. *It is advised that you always check with your medical doctor before starting any new exercise program or change in diet.*

LOST TEMPLE FITNESS & REHAB

INTRODUCTION

DIABETES
See Section for Specific TOC

REFERENCES

HOME EXERCISE PROGRAM
See Section for Specific TOC

Benefits / Before Starting a Routine

Averages – Body Temperature, Respiration, Blood Pressure, Heart Rate

How to Monitor Intensity of Heart Rate

Temperature – Heat and Cold

Dehydration

Altitude

Warm up/cool down

Duration, Frequency, Intensity & Movement Patterns

Breathing –Diaphragmatic, Purse lipped and with Resistance training

Anatomy - Positions, Directions, Muscle - joint action, Skeletal ROM

Equipment that may be needed

Self-Tests – Prior to starting program

Worksheets – Exercise Section/Numbers, Reps, Sets, x-day and Holds

Exercise Section/Numbers and Notes

Calorie

REFERENCES

Diabetes Table of Contents

Information from NIH – National Institute of Diabetes, Digestive and Kidney Diseases unless otherwise indicated.

Quick Summary of Section

Some Definitions

Ketones *WebMD*	Everyone has ketones, whether you have diabetes or not. • Ketones are chemicals made in your liver. • You produce them when you don't have enough insulin in your body to turn sugar (or glucose) into energy. • You need another source, so your body uses fat instead. Your liver turns this fat into ketones, a type of acid, and sends them into your bloodstream. • Your muscles and other tissues can then use them for fuel. For a person without diabetes, this process doesn't become an issue. • When you have diabetes, however, you can build up too many ketones in your blood -- and too many ketones can become life-threatening. 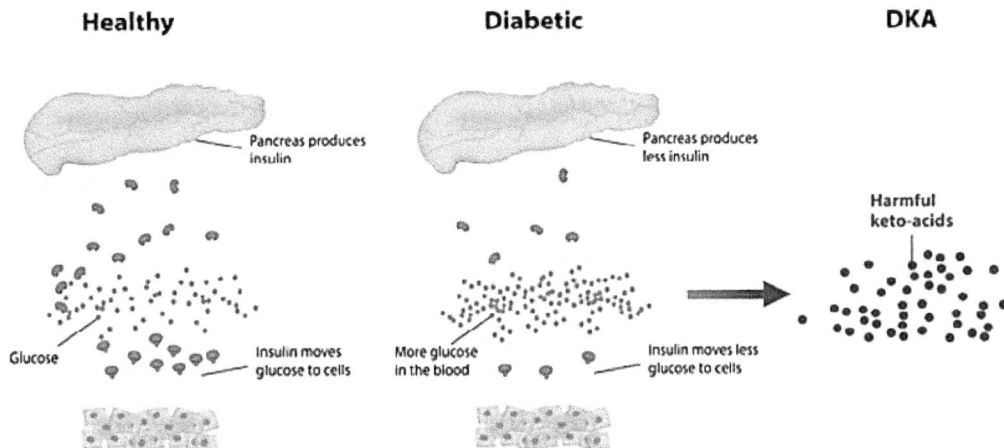
Diabetic Ketoacidosis (DKA) *MedLine Plus*	**Diabetic ketoacidosis (DKA)** is a life-threatening problem that affects people with diabetes. It occurs when the body starts breaking down fat at a rate that is much too fast. The liver processes the fat into a fuel called ketones, which causes the blood to become acidic. **Causes** DKA happens when the signal from insulin in the body is so low that: • Glucose (blood sugar) can't go into cells to be used as a fuel source. • The liver makes a huge amount of blood sugar. • Fat is broken down too rapidly for the body to process. The fat is broken down by the liver into a fuel called ketones. • *Ketones* are normally produced when the body breaks down fat after a long time between meals. • When ketones are produced too quickly and build up in the blood and urine, they can be toxic by making the blood acidic. This condition is known as *ketoacidosis*. DKA is sometimes the first sign of *type 1 diabetes* in people who have not yet been diagnosed. • It can also occur in someone who has already been diagnosed with type 1 diabetes. • Infection, injury, a serious illness, missing doses of insulin shots, or surgery can lead to DKA in people with type 1 diabetes. People with *type 2 diabetes* can also develop DKA, but it is less common and less severe. • It is usually triggered by prolonged uncontrolled blood sugar, missing doses of medicines, or a severe illness or infection.

Hyperosmolar Hyperglycemic State (HHS) *Cleveland Clinic*	**What is hyperosmolar hyperglycemic state?** • Hyperosmolar hyperglycemic state (HHS) is a life-threatening complication of diabetes — mainly Type 2 diabetes. • HHS happens when your blood glucose (sugar) levels are too high for a long period, leading to severe dehydration and confusion. • HHS requires immediate medical treatment. Without treatment, it can be fatal.

What's the difference between DKA and HHS?

Diabetes-related ketoacidosis (DKA) and hyperosmolar hyperglycemic state (HHS) are both life-threatening diabetes complications related to high blood sugar (hyperglycemia), but they're different conditions.

- *DKA* happens when your body doesn't have enough insulin. Your body needs insulin to turn glucose, your body's go-to source of fuel, into energy.
  - If there's no insulin or not enough insulin, your body starts breaking down fat for energy instead.
  - As your body breaks down fat, it releases ketones into your bloodstream.
  - Ketones cause your blood to become acidic, which is life-threatening.

- *HHS* happens when very high blood sugar leads to severe dehydration and highly concentrated blood (high osmolality), which are life-threatening.
  - HHS also involves a lack of insulin, but the person usually still produces enough insulin to prevent the production of ketones.
  - In addition, there's usually an underlying condition, such as an infection, that's also contributing to the high blood sugar.

DKA	HHS
Type I DM	Type II DM
Blood Sugar > 250 mg/dl	Blood Sugar > 600 mg/dl
Acetone Breath	No Fruity Smell
Ketones in Urine	Minimal or no Ketones
pH < 7.35	Normal pH, no Acidosis
Kussmaul's Respirations	Shallow Breath
Develops Quickly	Develops Slowly
Nausea, Vomiting, Abdominal Pain	Severely Altetred LOC
	Profound Dehydration

The main difference between DKA and HHS is that DKA involves ketones and blood acidity; HHS doesn't.
- The two complications have similar symptoms, including intense thirst, frequent urination and mental status changes.
  Cleveland Clinic

Insulin	**What is insulin?**
	Insulin is a hormone made by the pancreas that helps glucose in your blood enter cells in your muscle, fat, and liver, where it's used for energy.

- Glucose comes from the food you eat.
- The liver also makes glucose in times of need, such as when you're fasting.
- When blood glucose, also called blood sugar, levels rise after you eat, your pancreas releases insulin into the blood.
- Insulin then lowers blood glucose to keep it in the normal range.

Type 1 diabetes

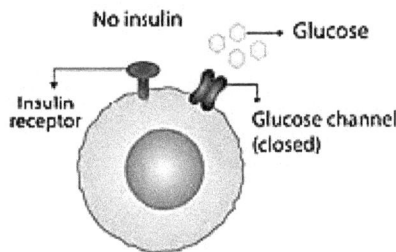

No insulin
→ Glucose

Insulin receptor

Glucose channel (closed)

Pancreas fails to produce insulin

Type 2 diabetes

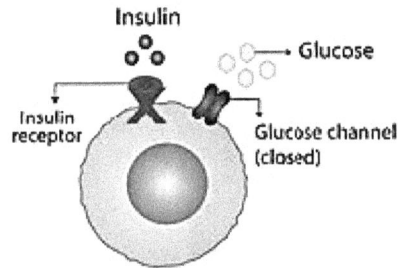

Insulin
→ Glucose

Insulin receptor

Glucose channel (closed)

Cells fail to respond to circulating insulin

What is insulin resistance?

Insulin resistance is when cells in your muscles, fat, and liver don't respond well to insulin and can't easily take up glucose from your blood.

- As a result, your pancreas makes more insulin to help glucose enter your cells.
- As long as your pancreas can make enough insulin to overcome your cells' weak response to insulin, your blood glucose levels will stay in the healthy range.

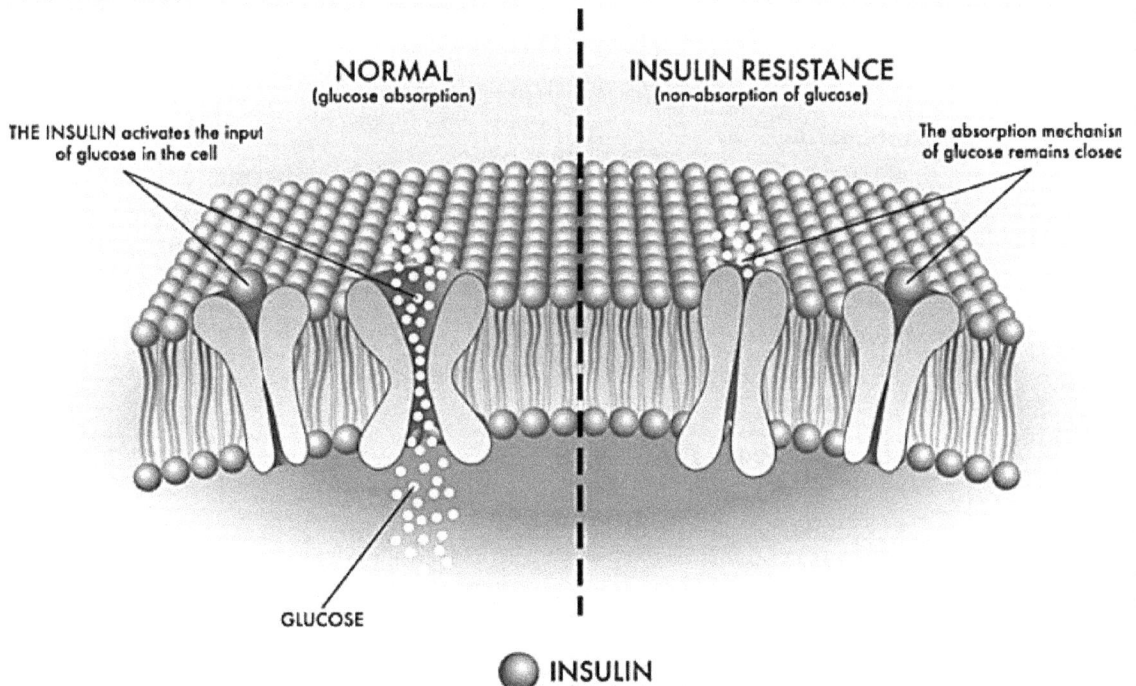

NORMAL
(glucose absorption)

INSULIN RESISTANCE
(non-absorption of glucose)

THE INSULIN activates the input of glucose in the cell

The absorption mechanism of glucose remains closed

GLUCOSE

INSULIN

Diabetes

What is Diabetes?	• Diabetes is a disease that occurs when your blood glucose, also called blood sugar, is too high. Blood glucose is your main source of energy and comes from the food you eat. Insulin, a hormone made by the pancreas, helps glucose from food get into your cells to be used for energy.
	• Sometimes your body doesn't make enough—or any—insulin or doesn't use insulin well. Glucose then stays in your blood and doesn't reach your cells.
	• Over time, having too much glucose in your blood can cause health problems. Although diabetes has no cure, you can take steps to manage your diabetes and stay healthy.
	• Sometimes people call diabetes "a touch of sugar" or "borderline diabetes." These terms suggest that someone doesn't really have diabetes or has a less serious case.

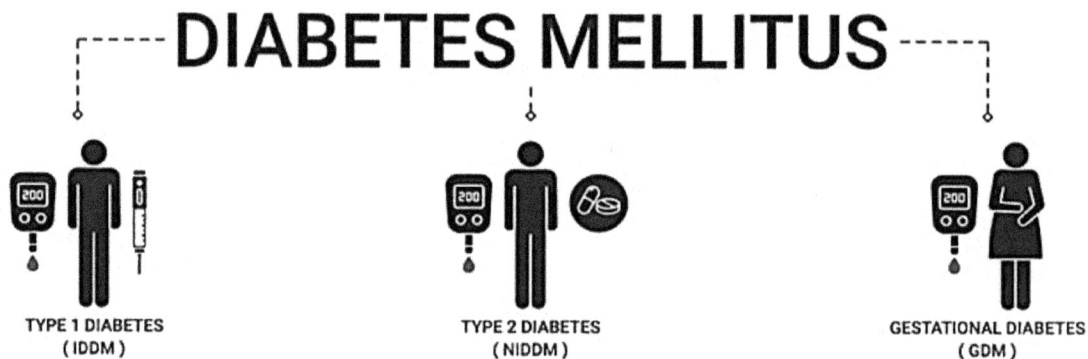

DIABETES MELLITUS

| TYPE 1 DIABETES (IDDM) | TYPE 2 DIABETES (NIDDM) | GESTATIONAL DIABETES (GDM) |

Types of Diabetes	*Type 1 diabetes*
	• If you have type 1 diabetes, your body does not make insulin. Your immune system attacks and destroys the cells in your pancreas that make insulin.
	• Type 1 diabetes is usually diagnosed in children and young adults, although it can appear at any age.
	• People with type 1 diabetes need to take insulin every day to stay alive.
	Type 2 diabetes
	• If you have type 2 diabetes, your body does not make or use insulin well.
	• You can develop type 2 diabetes at any age, even during childhood. However, this type of diabetes occurs most often in middle-aged and older people.
	• Type 2 is the most common type of diabetes.
	Gestational diabetes
	• Gestational diabetes develops in some women when they are pregnant.
	• Most of the time, this type of diabetes goes away after the baby is born. However, if you've had gestational diabetes, you have a greater chance of developing type 2 diabetes later in life.
	• Sometimes diabetes diagnosed during pregnancy is actually type 2 diabetes.
	Other types of diabetes
	• Less common types include diabetes insipidus, monogenic diabetes and cystic fibrosis-related diabetes.
Health Problems Related to Diabetes	Over time, high blood glucose leads to problems such as: • Heart disease • Stroke • Kidney disease • Eye problems • Dental disease • Nerve damage • Foot problems

Symptoms	Symptoms of diabetes include:
	• Increased thirst and urination • Increased hunger • Fatigue • Blurred vision • Numbness or tingling in the feet or hands • Sores that do not heal • Unexplained weight loss

DIABETES SYMPTOMS

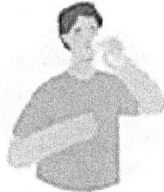 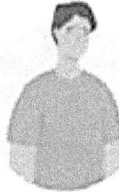 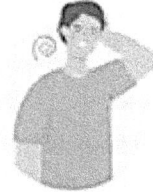 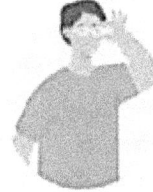 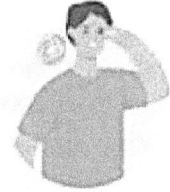

THIRST   WEAKNESS   DIZZINESS   BLURRY VISION   CONFUSION

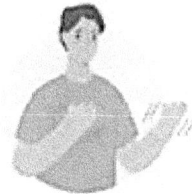 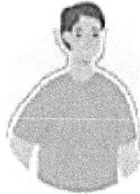 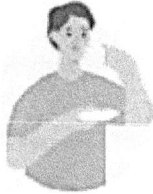 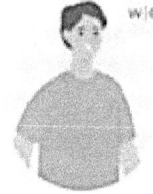 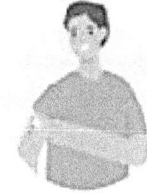

TINGLING HANDS   WEIGHT LOSS   ALWAYS HUNGRY   FREQUENT URINATION   WOUNDS THAT
OR FEET   WON'T HEAL

• Symptoms of type 1 diabetes can start quickly, in a matter of weeks.
• Symptoms of type 2 diabetes often develop slowly—over the course of several years—and can be so mild that you might not even notice them.
   o Many people with type 2 diabetes have no symptoms.
• Some people do not find out they have the disease until they have diabetes-related health problems, such as blurred vision or heart trouble.

Other Causes
 	
*See Type 1,
Type 2
and
Gestational
sections for
specific causes*
	Genetic mutations
	- *Monogenic diabetes* is caused by mutations, or changes, in a single gene. These changes are usually passed through families, but sometimes the gene mutation happens on its own. Most of these gene mutations cause diabetes by making the pancreas less able to make insulin.
	  - The most common types of monogenic diabetes are neonatal diabetes and maturity-onset diabetes of the young (MODY).
	  - Neonatal diabetes occurs in the first 6 months of life. Doctors usually diagnose MODY during adolescence or early adulthood, but sometimes the disease is not diagnosed until later in life.
	- **Cystic fibrosis** produces thick mucus that causes scarring in the pancreas. This scarring can prevent the pancreas from making enough insulin.
	- **Hemochromatosis** causes the body to store too much iron. If the disease is not treated, iron can build up in and damage the pancreas and other organs.
	
	Hormonal diseases
	Some hormonal diseases cause the body to produce too much of certain hormones, which sometimes cause insulin resistance and diabetes.
	- *Cushing's syndrome* occurs when the body produces too much cortisol—often called the "stress hormone."
	- *Acromegaly* occurs when the body produces too much growth hormone.
	- *Hyperthyroidism* occurs when the thyroid gland produces too much thyroid hormone.
	
	Damage to or removal of the pancreas
	- *Pancreatitis, pancreatic cancer, and trauma* can all harm the beta cells or make them less able to produce insulin, resulting in diabetes.
	- If the damaged pancreas is removed, diabetes will occur due to the loss of the beta cells.
	
	Medicines
	Sometimes certain medicines can harm beta cells or disrupt the way insulin works. These include
	- Niacin, a type of vitamin B3
	- Certain types of diuretics, also called water pills
	- Anti-seizure drugs
	- Psychiatric drugs
	- Drugs to treat human immunodeficiency virus (HIV)
	- Pentamidine, a drug used to treat a type of pneumonia
	- Glucocorticoids—medicines used to treat inflammatory illnesses such as rheumatoid arthritis , asthma , lupus , and ulcerative colitis
	- Anti-rejection medicines, used to help stop the body from rejecting a transplanted organ
	- Statins, which are medicines to reduce LDL ("bad") cholesterol levels, can slightly increase the chance that you'll develop diabetes.
	  - However, statins help protect you from heart disease and stroke.
	  - For this reason, the strong benefits of taking statins outweigh the small chance that you could develop diabetes.

	Type 1
What is Type 1 Diabetes? **Who is More Likely to Develop Type 1 Diabetes?**	Diabetes occurs when your blood glucose, also called blood sugar, is too high. • Blood glucose is your main source of energy and comes mainly from the food you eat. • Insulin, a hormone made by the pancreas, helps the glucose in your blood get into your cells to be used for energy. • Another hormone, glucagon, works with insulin to control blood glucose levels. • In most people with type 1 diabetes, the body's immune system, which normally fights infection, attacks and destroys the cells in the pancreas that make insulin. As a result, your pancreas stops making insulin. • Without insulin, glucose can't get into your cells and your blood glucose rises above normal. • People with type 1 diabetes need to take insulin every day to stay alive. **Type 1 Diabetes** Glucose — Glucose is extracted from food in the stomach. Insulin — The pancreas produces little or no insulin. Pancreas An increased amount of glucose remains in the blood. Muscles and organs are unable to use glucose due low insulin. *Who is more likely to develop type 1 diabetes?* • Type 1 diabetes typically occurs in children and young adults, although it can appear at any age. • Having a parent or sibling with the disease may increase your chance of developing type 1 diabetes. • In the United States, about 5 percent of people with diabetes have type 1.
Causes	• Type 1 diabetes occurs when your immune system, the body's system for fighting infection, attacks and destroys the insulin-producing beta cells of the pancreas. • Scientists think type 1 diabetes is caused by genes and environmental factors, such as viruses, that might trigger the disease. • Studies such as Trial Net are working to pinpoint causes of type 1 diabetes and possible ways to prevent or slow the disease.

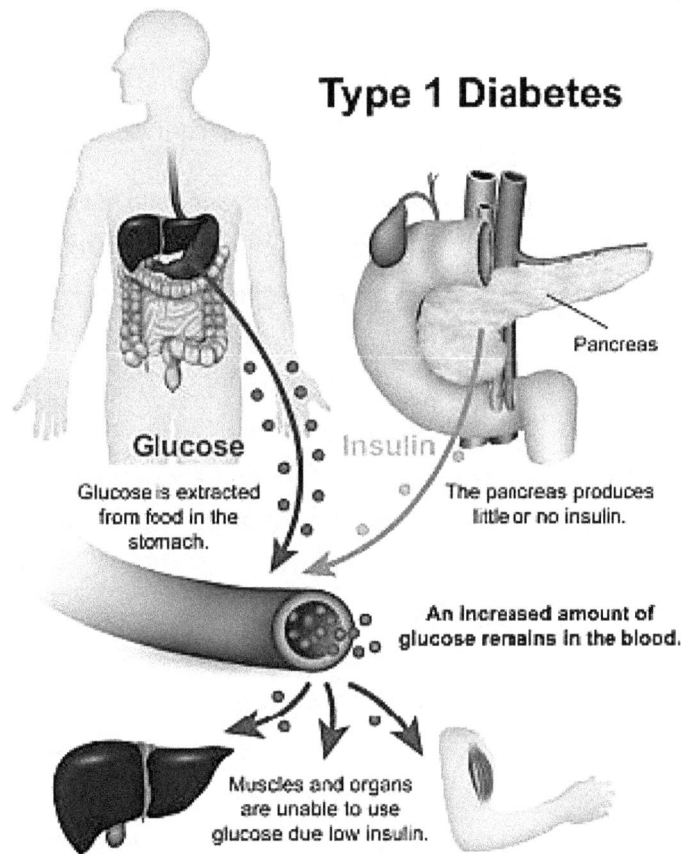

Symptoms	Symptoms of type 1 diabetes are serious and usually happen quickly, over a few days to weeks. Symptoms can include: • Increased thirst and urination • Increased hunger • Blurred vision • Fatigue • Unexplained weight loss • Sometimes the first symptoms of type 1 diabetes are signs of a life-threatening condition called diabetic ketoacidosis (DKA). Some symptoms of DKA include: • Breath that smells fruity • Dry or flushed skin • Nausea or vomiting • Stomach pain • Trouble breathing • Trouble paying attention or feeling confused ***DKA is serious and dangerous.*** If you or your child have symptoms of DKA, contact your health care professional right away, or go to the nearest hospital emergency room.

Health Problems Related to Diabetes	Over time, high blood glucose leads to problems such as: • Heart disease • Stroke • Kidney disease • Eye problems • Dental disease • Nerve damage • Foot problems • Depression • Sleep apnea If you have type 1 diabetes, you can help prevent or delay the health problems of diabetes by managing your blood glucose, blood pressure, and cholesterol, and following your self-care plan.

Medicines
 	
Also see: *Insulin, Medicines, & Other Diabetes Treatments*
	• If you have type 1 diabetes, you must take insulin because your body no longer makes this hormone.
	   ○ Different types of insulin start to work at different speeds, and the effects of each last a different length of time.
	   ○ You may need to use more than one type.
	   ○ You can take insulin a number of ways. Common options include a needle and syringe, insulin pen, or insulin pump.
	• Some people who have trouble reaching their blood glucose targets with insulin alone also might need to take another type of diabetes medicine that works with insulin, such as pramlintide.
	   ○ *Pramlintide*, given by injection, helps keep blood glucose levels from going too high after eating.
	   ○ Few people with type 1 diabetes take pramlintide, however.
	   ○ The NIH has recently funded a large research study to test use of pramlintide along with insulin and glucagon in people with type 1 diabetes.
	• Another diabetes medicine, *metformin*, may help decrease the amount of insulin you need to take, but more studies are needed to confirm this.
	• Researchers are also studying other diabetes pills that people with type 1 diabetes might take along with insulin.
	
	Hypoglycemia, or low blood sugar, can occur if you take insulin but don't match your dose with your food or physical activity.
	• Severe hypoglycemia can be dangerous and needs to be treated right away.
	
	Blood Glucose Level

Other Ways to Manage
 	
National Institute of Diabetes and Digestive & Kidney Diseases (NIDDK)
	Along with insulin and any other medicines you use, you can manage your diabetes by taking care of yourself each day.
	
	• Following your diabetes meal plan, being physically active, and checking your blood glucose often are some of the ways you can take care of yourself.
	• Work with your health care team to come up with a diabetes care plan that works for you. If you are planning a pregnancy with diabetes, try to get your blood glucose levels in your target range before you get pregnant.
	
	 TYPE 1 DIABETES
	MANAGEMENT
	
	blood glucose level monitoring lifelong insulin injections
	
	regular physical activity healthy diet
	Other treatment options:
	
	• The National Institute of Diabetes and Digestive and Kidney Diseases (NIDDK) has played an important role in developing "artificial pancreas" technology.
	   o An artificial pancreas replaces manual blood glucose testing and the use of insulin shots. A single system monitors blood glucose levels around the clock and provides insulin or a combination of insulin and glucagon automatically.
	   o The system can also be monitored remotely, for example by parents or medical staff.
	• In 2016, the U.S. Food and Drug Administration approved a type of artificial pancreas system called a hybrid closed-loop system.
	   o This system tests your glucose level every 5 minutes throughout the day and night through a continuous glucose monitor and automatically gives you the right amount of basal insulin, a long-acting insulin, through a separate insulin pump.
	   o You still need to manually adjust the amount of insulin the pump delivers at mealtimes and when you need a correction dose.
	   o You also will need to test your blood with a glucose meter several times a day.
	• The continuous glucose monitor sends information through a software program called a control algorithm.
	   o Based on your glucose level, the algorithm tells the insulin pump how much insulin to deliver. The software program could be installed on the pump or another device such as a cell phone or computer.
	• The devices may also help people with type 2 diabetes and gestational diabetes.
	• NIDDK is also supporting research into pancreatic islet transplantation—an experimental treatment for hard-to-control type 1 diabetes.
	   o Pancreatic islets are clusters of cells in the pancreas that make insulin. Type 1 diabetes attacks these cells.
	   o A pancreatic islet transplant replaces destroyed islets with new ones that make and release insulin. This procedure takes islets from the pancreas of an organ donor and transfers them to a person with type 1 diabetes.
	   o Because researchers are still studying pancreatic islet transplantation, the procedure is only available to people enrolled in a study.

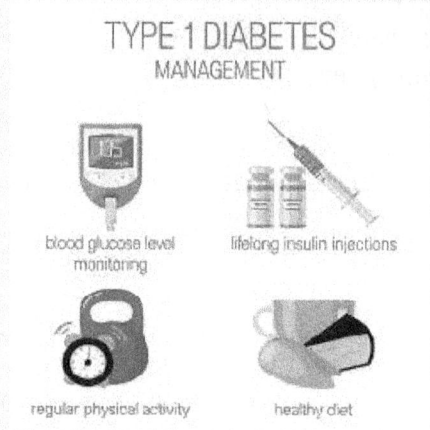

	Type 2
What is Type 2 Diabetes?	• Type 2 diabetes, the most common type of diabetes, is a disease that occurs when your blood glucose, also called blood sugar, is too high. • Blood glucose is your main source of energy and comes mainly from the food you eat. Insulin, a hormone made by the pancreas, helps glucose get into your cells to be used for energy. • In type 2 diabetes, your body doesn't make enough insulin or doesn't use insulin well. ○ Too much glucose then stays in your blood, and not enough reaches your cells. 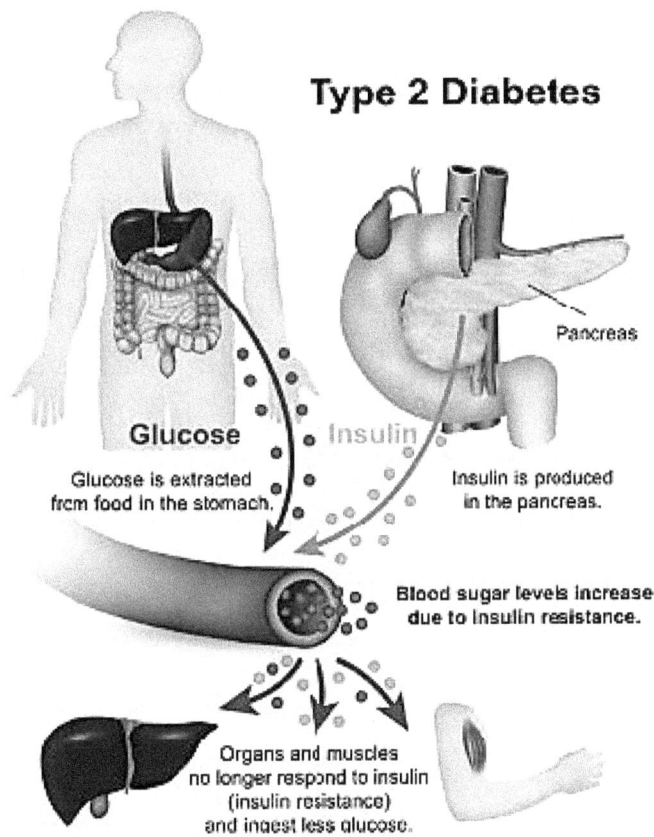

Type 2 Diabetes

Glucose

Glucose is extracted from food in the stomach.

Insulin

Insulin is produced in the pancreas.

Pancreas

Blood sugar levels increase due to insulin resistance.

Organs and muscles no longer respond to insulin (insulin resistance) and ingest less glucose.

Causes & Risks	Your chances of developing type 2 diabetes depend on a combination of risk factors such as your genes and lifestyle. • Although you can't change risk factors such as family history, age, or ethnicity, you can change lifestyle risk factors around eating, physical activity, and weight. • These lifestyle changes can affect your chances of developing type 2 diabetes. ***You are more likely to develop type 2 diabetes if you:*** • Are overweight or obese • Are age 45 or older • Have a family history of diabetes • Are African American, Alaska Native, American Indian, Asian American, Hispanic/Latino, Native Hawaiian, or Pacific Islander • Have high blood pressure • Have a low level of HDL ("good") cholesterol, or a high level of triglycerides • Have a history of gestational diabetes or gave birth to a baby weighing 9 pounds or more • Are not physically active • Have a history of heart disease or stroke • Have depression NIH external link • Have polycystic ovary syndrome NIH external link, also called PCOS • Have acanthosis nigricans—dark, thick, and velvety skin around your neck or armpits **CAUSES OF TYPE 2 DIABETES** 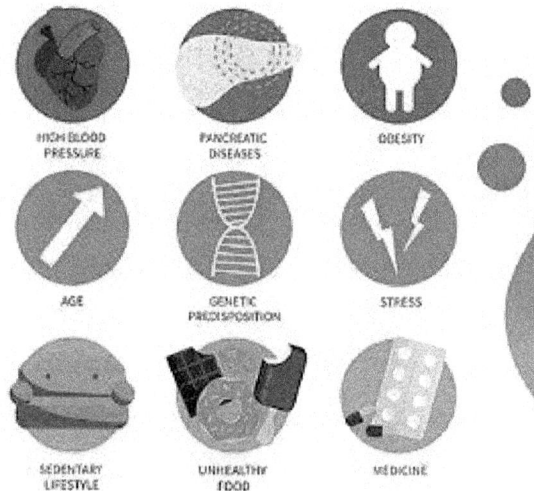 ***Overweight, obesity, and physical inactivity*** • You are more likely to develop type 2 diabetes if you are not physically active and are overweight or obese. Extra weight sometimes causes insulin resistance and is common in people with type 2 diabetes. • The location of body fat also makes a difference. Extra belly fat is linked to insulin resistance, type 2 diabetes, and heart and blood vessel disease. • To see if your weight puts you at risk for type 2 diabetes, check out these Body Mass Index (BMI) charts. ***Insulin resistance*** • Type 2 diabetes usually begins with insulin resistance, a condition in which muscle, liver, and fat cells do not use insulin well. As a result, your body needs more insulin to help glucose enter cells. • At first, the pancreas makes more insulin to keep up with the added demand. • Over time, the pancreas can't make enough insulin, and blood glucose levels rise.

Symptoms Also see *Diabetic Neuropathy*	Symptoms of diabetes include: • Increased thirst and urination • Increased hunger • Feeling tired • Blurred vision • Numbness or tingling in the feet or hands • Sores that do not heal • Unexplained weight loss Symptoms of type 2 diabetes often develop slowly—over the course of several years—and can be so mild that you might not even notice them. • Many people have no symptoms. Some people do not find out they have the disease until they have diabetes-related health problems, such as blurred vision or heart disease.
Health Problems Related to Diabetes Also see *Diabetes and Foot Problems*	Following a good diabetes care plan can help protect against many diabetes-related health problems. However, if not managed, diabetes can lead to problems such as • Heart disease and stroke • Nerve damage • Kidney disease • Foot problems • Eye disease • Gum disease and other dental problems • Sexual and bladder problems • Many people with type 2 diabetes also have nonalcoholic fatty liver disease (NAFLD). Losing weight if you are overweight or obese can improve NAFLD. • Diabetes is also linked to other health problems such as sleep apnea, depression, some types of cancer, and dementia.
Ways to Manage Also see *Insulin, Medicines, & Other Diabetes Treatments*	Managing your blood glucose, blood pressure, and cholesterol, and quitting smoking if you smoke, are important ways to manage your type 2 diabetes. • Lifestyle changes that include planning healthy meals, limiting calories if you are overweight, and being physically active are also part of managing your diabetes. • So is taking any prescribed medicines. • Work with your health care team to create a diabetes care plan that works for you. ***What medicines do I need to treat my type 2 diabetes?*** • Along with following your diabetes care plan, you may need diabetes medicines, which may include pills or medicines you inject under your skin, such as insulin. • Over time, you may need more than one diabetes medicine to manage your blood glucose. • Even if you don't take insulin, you may need it at special times, such as during pregnancy or if you are in the hospital. • You also may need medicines for high blood pressure, high cholesterol, or other conditions.

Body Mass Index (BMI)	To see if your weight puts you at risk for type 2 diabetes, find your height in the Body Mass Index (BMI) charts below. If your weight is equal to or more than the weight listed, you have a greater chance of developing the disease.

If you are NOT Asian American or Pacific Islander		If you are Asian American		If you are Pacific Islander	
At-risk BMI ≥ 25		At-risk BMI ≥ 23		At-risk BMI ≥ 26	
Height	Weight	Height	Weight	Height	Weight
4'10"	119	4'10"	110	4'10"	124
4'11"	124	4'11"	114	4'11"	128
5'0"	128	5'0"	118	5'0"	133
5'1"	132	5'1"	122	5'1"	137
5'2"	136	5'2"	126	5'2"	142
5'3"	141	5'3"	130	5'3"	146
5'4"	145	5'4"	134	5'4"	151
5'5"	150	5'5"	138	5'5"	156
5'6"	155	5'6"	142	5'6"	161
5'7"	159	5'7"	146	5'7"	166
5'8"	164	5'8"	151	5'8"	171
5'9"	169	5'9"	155	5'9"	176
5'10"	174	5'10"	160	5'10"	181
5'11"	179	5'11"	165	5'11"	186
6'0"	184	6'0"	169	6'0"	191
6'1"	189	6'1"	174	6'1"	197
6'2"	194	6'2"	179	6'2"	202
6'3"	200	6'3"	184	6'3"	208
6'4"	205	6'4"	189	6'4"	213

Prevention	*How can I lower my chances of developing type 2 diabetes?*
	 Research such as the Diabetes Prevention Program shows that you can do a lot to reduce your chances of developing type 2 diabetes. Here are some things you can change to lower your risk:
	 • **Lose weight** and keep it off.
	   ○ You may be able to prevent or delay diabetes by losing 5 to 7 percent of your starting weight. For instance, if you weigh 200 pounds, your goal would be to lose about 10 to 14 pounds.
	 • **Move more**. Get at least 30 minutes of physical activity 5 days a week.
	   ○ If you have not been active, talk with your health care professional about which activities are best. Start slowly to build up to your goal.
	 • **Eat healthy foods** most of the time.
	   ○ Eat smaller portions to reduce the amount of calories you eat each day and help you lose weight.
	   ○ Choosing foods with less fat is another way to reduce calories. Drink water instead of sweetened beverages.
	
	 Ask your health care professional about what other changes you can make to prevent or delay type 2 diabetes. Most often, your best chance for preventing type 2 diabetes is to make lifestyle changes that work for you long term.

Gestational Diabetes

What is Gestational Diabetes?	• Gestational diabetes is a type of diabetes that develops during pregnancy. Diabetes means your blood glucose, also called blood sugar, is too high. Too much glucose in your blood is not good for you or your baby. • Usually, gestational diabetes has no symptoms. If you do have symptoms, they may be mild, such as being thirstier than normal or having to urinate more often. • Gestational diabetes is usually diagnosed in the 24th to 28th week of pregnancy. Managing your gestational diabetes can help you and your baby stay healthy. You can protect your own and your baby's health by taking action right away to manage your blood glucose levels. 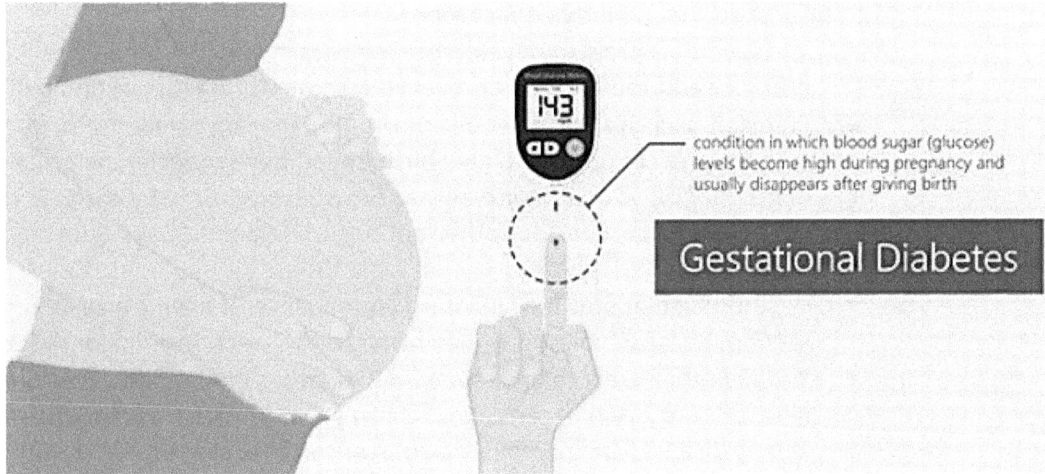 *Insulin resistance* • Hormones produced by the placenta contribute to insulin resistance, which occurs in all women during late pregnancy. • Most pregnant women can produce enough insulin to overcome insulin resistance, but some cannot. • Gestational diabetes occurs when the pancreas can't make enough insulin. • As with type 2 diabetes, extra weight is linked to gestational diabetes. Women who are overweight or obese may already have insulin resistance when they become pregnant. • Gaining too much weight during pregnancy may also be a factor.

How can Gestational Diabetes Affect My Baby and/or Me?	High blood glucose levels during pregnancy can cause problems for your baby, such as • Being born too early • Weighing too much, which can make delivery difficult and injure your baby • Having low blood glucose, also called hypoglycemia, right after birth • Having breathing problems • High blood glucose also can increase the chance that you will have a miscarriage or a stillborn baby. Stillborn means the baby dies in the womb during the second half of pregnancy. • Your baby also will be more likely to become overweight and develop type 2 diabetes as he or she gets older. *How can gestational diabetes affect me?* • You are more likely to develop **preeclampsia,** which is when you develop high blood pressure and too much protein in your urine during the second half of pregnancy. • Preeclampsia can cause serious or life-threatening problems for you and your baby. The only cure for preeclampsia is to give birth. If you have preeclampsia and have reached 37 weeks of pregnancy, your doctor may want to deliver your baby early. Before 37 weeks, you and your doctor may consider other options to help your baby develop as much as possible before he or she is born. • Gestational diabetes may increase your chance of having a cesarean section , also called a C-section, because your baby may be large. A C-section is major surgery. • You are more likely to develop type 2 diabetes later in life. Over time, having too much glucose in your blood can cause health problems such as diabetic retinopathy, heart disease, kidney disease, and nerve damage. You can take steps to help Hormonal changes, extra weight, and family history can contribute to gestational diabetes. 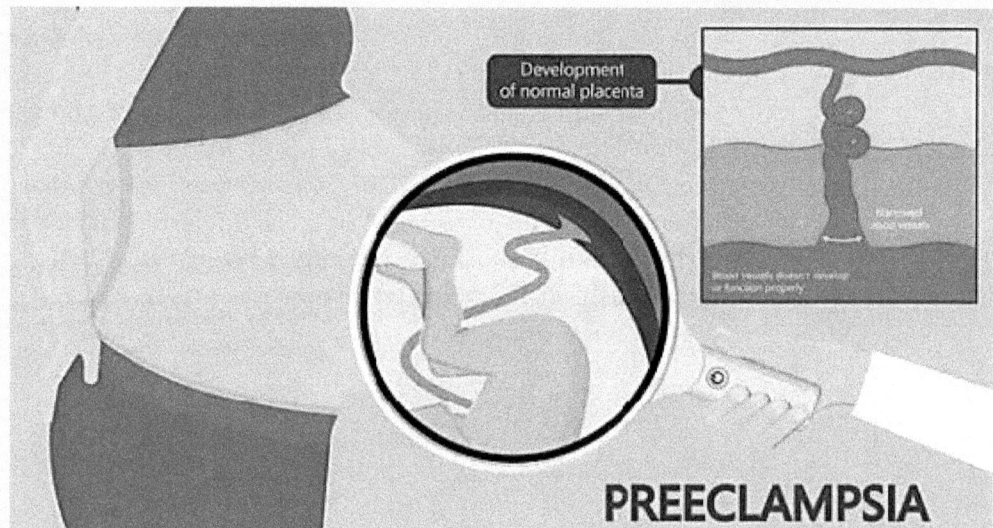 *Genes and family history:* • Having a family history of diabetes makes it more likely that a woman will develop gestational diabetes, which suggests that genes play a role. • Genes may also explain why the disorder occurs more often in African Americans, American Indians, Asians, and Hispanics/Latinas.

Causes	• Gestational diabetes occurs when your body can't make the extra insulin needed during pregnancy. Insulin, a hormone made in your pancreas, helps your body use glucose for energy and helps control your blood glucose levels.
	• During pregnancy, your body makes special hormones and goes through other changes, such as weight gain.
	    o Because of these changes, your body's cells don't use insulin well, a condition called insulin resistance.
	    o All pregnant women have some insulin resistance during late pregnancy.
	    o Most pregnant women can produce enough insulin to overcome insulin resistance, but some cannot.
	    o These women develop gestational diabetes.
	• Being overweight or obese is linked to gestational diabetes.
	    o Women who are overweight or obese may already have insulin resistance when they become pregnant.
	    o Gaining too much weight during pregnancy may also be a factor.
	• Having a family history of diabetes makes it more likely that a woman will develop gestational diabetes, which suggests that genes play a role.

Ways to Manage Also see *Insulin, Medicines, & Other Diabetes Treatments*	***Follow a healthy eating plan*** • Your health care team will help you make a healthy eating plan with food choices that are good for you and your baby. The plan will help you know which foods to eat, how much to eat, and when to eat. Food choices, amounts, and timing are all important in keeping your blood glucose levels in your target range. • If you're not eating enough or your blood glucose is too high, your body might make ketones. Ketones in your urine or blood mean your body is using fat for energy instead of glucose. Burning large amounts of fat instead of glucose can be harmful to your health and your baby's health. • Your doctor might recommend you test your urine or blood daily for ketones or when your blood glucose is above a certain level, such as 200. If your ketone levels are high, your doctor may suggest that you change the type or amount of food you eat, or you may need to change your meal or snack times. **TARGET BLOOD SUGAR LEVELS FOR PREGNANT WOMEN** **Pre-existing diabetes** *Fasting and before meal* **60-99** *After meal (1hr-2hr)* **100-129** *Amounts shown above mg/dL* **A1c** *less than* **6%** **Gestational diabetes** *Fasting and before meal* *less than* **99** *After meal (1hr-2hr)* *less than* **120**

Ways to Manage *Continued* Also see *Insulin, Medicines, & Other Diabetes Treatments*	***Be physically active*** • Physical activity can help you reach your target blood glucose levels. If your blood pressure or cholesterol levels are too high, being physically active can help you reach healthy levels. • Physical activity can also relieve stress, strengthen your heart and bones, improve muscle strength, and keep your joints flexible. • Being physically active will also help lower your chances of having type 2 diabetes in the future. Talk with your health care team about what activities are best for you during your pregnancy. • Aim for 30 minutes of activity 5 days of the week, even if you weren't active before your pregnancy. • If you are already active, tell your doctor what you do. Ask your doctor if you can continue some higher intensity activities, such as lifting weights or jogging. ***How will I know whether my blood glucose levels are on target?*** • Your health care team may ask you to use a blood glucose meter to check your blood glucose levels. • This device uses a small drop of blood from your finger to measure your blood glucose level. Your health care team can show you how to use your meter. Recommended daily target blood glucose levels for most women with gestational diabetes are: • Before meals, at bedtime, and overnight: 95 or less • 1 hour after eating: 140 or less • 2 hours after eating: 120 or less • Ask your doctor what targets are right for you. Your health care team may ask you to use a ***blood glucose meter*** to check your blood glucose levels. • You can keep track of your blood glucose levels using My Daily Blood Glucose Record (PDF, 45 KB). You can also use an electronic blood glucose tracking system on your computer or mobile device. • Record the results every time you check your blood glucose. Your blood glucose records can help you and your health care team decide whether your diabetes care plan is working. Take your tracker with you when you visit your health care team. ***How is gestational diabetes treated if diet and physical activity aren't enough?*** • If following your eating plan and being physically active aren't enough to keep your blood glucose levels in your target range, you may need insulin. • If you need to use ***insulin***, your health care team will show you how to give yourself insulin shots. Insulin will not harm your baby and is usually the first choice of diabetes medicine for gestational diabetes. • Researchers are studying the safety of the diabetes pills metformin and glyburide during pregnancy, but more long-term studies are needed. Talk with your health care professional about what treatment is right for you.

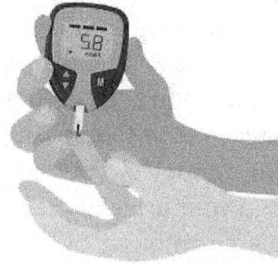

Insulin, Medicines & Other Diabetes Treatments

Possible Medicines for Diabetes	<ul><li>Taking insulin or other diabetes medicines is often part of treating diabetes. Along with healthy food choices and physical activity, medicine can help you manage the disease. Some other treatment options are also available.</li><li>The medicine you take will vary by your type of diabetes and how well the medicine controls your blood glucose levels, also called blood sugar.</li><li>Other factors, such as your other health conditions, medication costs, and your daily schedule may play a role in what diabetes medicine you take.</li></ul>

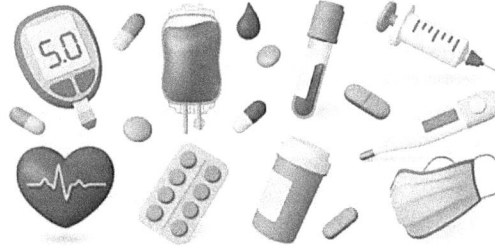

Type 1 diabetes

- If you have type 1 diabetes, you must take insulin because your pancreas does not make it. You will need to take insulin several times during the day, including when you eat and drink, to control your blood glucose level.
- There are different ways to take insulin. You can use a needle and syringe, an insulin pen, or an insulin pump. An artificial pancreas—also called an automated insulin delivery system—may be another option for some people.

Type 2 diabetes

- Some people with type 2 diabetes can control their blood glucose level by making lifestyle changes. These lifestyle changes include consuming healthy meals and beverages, limiting calories if they have overweight or obesity, and getting physical activity.
- Many people with type 2 diabetes need to take diabetes medicines as well. These medicines may include diabetes pills or medicines you inject, such as insulin.
- Over time, you may need more than one diabetes medicine to control your blood glucose level.
- Even if you do not take insulin, you may need it at special times, such as if you are pregnant or if you are in the hospital for treatment.

Gestational diabetes

- If you have gestational diabetes, you can manage your blood glucose level by following a healthy eating plan and doing a moderate-intensity physical activity, such as brisk walking for 150 minutes, each week.
- If consuming healthy food and beverages and getting regular physical activity aren't enough to keep your blood glucose level in your target range, a doctor will work with you and may recommend you take insulin. Insulin is safe to take while you are pregnant.

No matter what type of diabetes you have, taking diabetes medicines every day can feel like a burden sometimes.

- New medications and improved delivery systems can help make it easier to manage your blood glucose levels.
- Talk with your doctor to find out which medications and delivery systems will work best for you and fit into your lifestyle.

Different Types of Insulin	Several types of insulin are available. Each type starts to work at a different speed, known as "onset," and its effects last a different length of time, known as "duration." • Most types of insulin reach a peak, which is when they have the strongest effect. Then the effects of the insulin wear off over the next few hours or so.

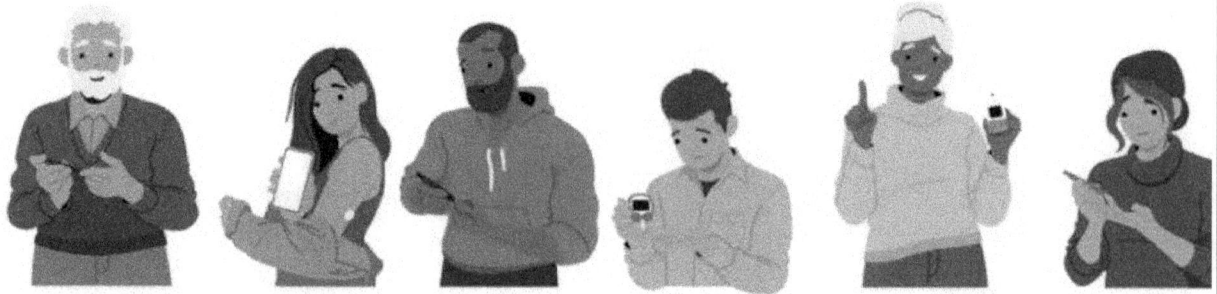

Types of Insulin and How They Work			
Insulin type	**How fast it starts to work (onset)**	**When it peaks**	**How long it lasts (duration)**
Rapid-acting/ ultra-rapid-acting	15 minutes	1 hour	2 to 4 hours (rapid) 5 to 7 hours (ultra)
Rapid-acting, inhaled	10-15 minutes	30 minutes	3 hours
Short-acting, also called regular	30 minutes	2 to 3 hours	3 to 6 hours
Intermediate-acting	2 to 4 hours after injection	4 to 12 hours	12 to 18 hours
Long-acting	2 hours	Does not peak	24 hours; some last longer
Ultra long acting	6 hours	Does not peak	36 hours or longer

The chart above gives averages. Follow your doctor's advice on when and how to take your insulin.

• Your doctor might also recommend premixed insulin, which is a mix of two types of insulin.

• Some types of insulin cost more than others, so talk with your doctor about your options if you're concerned about cost.

Source: *Insulin basics. American Diabetes Association website. Accessed 2022*

Insulin injection sites

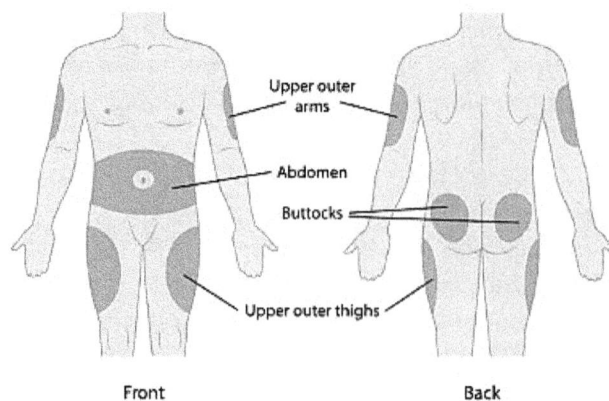

Upper outer arms

Abdomen

Buttocks

Upper outer thighs

Front   Back

Different Ways to Take Insulin	The way you take insulin may depend on your lifestyle, insurance plan, and preferences. You may decide that needles are not for you and prefer a different method. *Needle and syringe* • You can give yourself insulin shots using a needle and syringe. You draw up your dose of insulin from the vial—or bottle—through the needle into the syringe. Insulin works fastest when you inject it in your belly, but your doctor may recommend alternating the spot where you inject it. Injecting insulin in the same spot repeatedly could cause the tissue to harden, making it harder to take shots in that area over time. Other spots you can inject insulin include your thigh, buttocks, or upper arm, but it may take longer for the insulin to work from those areas. • Some people with diabetes who take insulin need 2 to 4 shots a day to reach their blood glucose targets. Others can take a single shot. Injection aids can help you give yourself the shots. *Pen* • An insulin pen looks like a writing pen but has a needle for its point. Some insulin pens come filled with insulin and are disposable. Others have room for an insulin cartridge that you insert and replace after use. Many people find insulin pens easier to use, but they cost more than needles and syringes. You may want to consider using an insulin pen if you find it hard to fill the syringe while holding the vial or cannot read the markings on the syringe. • Different pen types have features that can help with your injections. Some reusable pens have a memory function, which can recall dose amounts and timing. Other types of "connected" insulin pens can be programmed to calculate insulin doses and provide downloadable data reports, which can help you and your doctor adjust your insulin doses. *Pump* • An insulin pump is a small machine that gives you steady doses of insulin throughout the day. You wear one type of pump outside your body on a belt or in a pocket or pouch. The insulin pump connects to a small plastic tube and a very small needle. You insert the plastic tube with a needle under your skin, then take out the needle. The plastic tube will stay inserted for several days while attached to the insulin pump. The machine pumps insulin through the tube into your body 24 hours a day and can be programmed to give you more or less insulin based on your needs. You can also give yourself doses of insulin through the pump at mealtimes. • Another type of pump has no tubes. This pump attaches directly to your skin with a self-adhesive pad and is controlled by a hand-held device. The plastic tube and pump device are changed every several days. *Inhaler* • Another way to take insulin is by breathing powdered insulin into your mouth from an inhaler device. The insulin goes into your lungs and moves quickly into your blood. You may want to use an insulin inhaler to avoid using needles. Inhaled insulin is only for adults with type 1 or type 2 diabetes. Taking insulin with an inhaler is less common than using a needle and syringe. *Artificial pancreas* • An artificial pancreas is a system of three devices that work together to mimic how a healthy pancreas controls blood glucose in the body. • A continuous glucose monitor (CGM) tracks blood glucose levels every few minutes using a small sensor inserted under the skin that is held in place with an adhesive pad. • The CGM wirelessly sends the information to a program on a smartphone or an insulin infusion pump. The program calculates how much insulin you need. • The insulin infusion pump will adjust how much insulin is given from minute to minute to help keep your blood glucose level in your target range. • An artificial pancreas is mainly used to help people with type 1 diabetes. *Jet injector* • This device sends a fine spray of insulin into the skin at high pressure instead of using a needle to deliver the insulin.

Oral and Injectable Medicines Treat Type 2 Diabetes	• You may need medicines along with healthy eating and physical activity habits to manage your type 2 diabetes. You can take many diabetes medicines by mouth. These medicines are called oral medicines. • Most people with type 2 diabetes start medical treatment with metformin pills. Metformin also comes as a liquid. Metformin lowers the amount of glucose that your liver makes and helps your body use insulin better. This drug may help you lose a small amount of weight. • Other oral medicines act in different ways to lower blood glucose levels. You may need to add another diabetes medicine after a while or use a combination treatment. Combining two or three kinds of diabetes medicines can lower blood glucose levels more than taking just one. *Injectable medicines* • Besides insulin, other types of injected medicines are available. These medicines help keep your blood glucose level from going too high after you eat. They may make you feel less hungry and help you lose some weight. Other injectable medicines are not substitutes for insulin.
Side Effects of Diabetes Medicines	Side effects are problems that result from a medicine. Some diabetes medicines can cause hypoglycemia, also called low blood glucose, if you don't balance your medicines with food and activity. Ask your doctor whether your diabetes medicine can cause hypoglycemia or other side effects, such as upset stomach and weight gain. Take your diabetes medicines as your health care professional has instructed you, to help prevent side effects and diabetes problems.
Other Treatment Options	*Bariatric surgery* • Also called weight-loss surgery or metabolic surgery, bariatric surgery may help some people with obesity and type 2 diabetes lose a large amount of weight and regain normal blood glucose levels. Some people with diabetes may no longer need their diabetes medicine after bariatric surgery. • Whether and for how long blood glucose levels improve seems to vary by the patient, type of weight-loss surgery, and amount of weight the person loses. Other factors include how long someone has had diabetes and whether or not the person uses insulin. *Artificial Pancreas* • The NIDDK has played an important role in developing "artificial pancreas" technology. An artificial pancreas replaces manual blood glucose testing and the use of insulin shots or a pump. A single system monitors blood glucose levels around the clock and provides insulin or a combination of insulin and a second hormone, glucagon, automatically. The system can also be monitored remotely, for example by parents or medical staff. • In 2016, the FDA approved a type of artificial pancreas system called a hybrid closed-loop system. This system tests your glucose level every 5 minutes throughout the day and night, and automatically gives you the right amount of insulin. • You still need to manually adjust the amount of insulin the pump delivers at mealtimes. But, the artificial pancreas may free you from some of the daily tasks needed to keep your blood glucose stable—or help you sleep through the night without the need to wake and test your glucose or take medicine. • The hybrid closed-loop system is expected to be available in the U.S. in 2017. Talk with your health care provider about whether this system might be right for you.

Diabetic Neuropathy

Also see *Peripheral Neuropathy*	Diabetic neuropathy is nerve damage that is caused by diabetes. Nerves are bundles of special tissues that carry signals between your brain and other parts of your body. The signals: • Send information about how things feel • Move your body parts • Control body functions such as digestion **Types of diabetic neuropathy include the following:** ***Peripheral neuropathy*** • Peripheral neuropathy is nerve damage that typically affects the feet and legs and sometimes affects the hands and arms. *(see peripheral neuropathy in next section)* ***Autonomic neuropathy*** • Autonomic neuropathy is damage to nerves that control your internal organs. Autonomic neuropathy can lead to problems with your heart rate and blood pressure, digestive system, bladder, sex organs, sweat glands, eyes, and ability to sense hypoglycemia. ***Focal neuropathy*** • Focal neuropathies are conditions in which you typically have damage to single nerves, most often in your hand, head, torso, and leg. ***Proximal neuropathy*** • Proximal neuropathy is a rare and disabling type of nerve damage in your hip, buttock, or thigh. This type of nerve damage typically affects one side of your body and may rarely spread to the other side. Proximal neuropathy often causes severe pain and may lead to significant weight loss.
Who is Most Likely to Get Diabetic Neuropathy?	If you have diabetes, your chance of developing nerve damage caused by diabetes increases the older you get and the longer you have diabetes. Managing your diabetes is an important part of preventing health problems such as diabetic neuropathy. You are also more likely to develop nerve damage if you have diabetes and: • Are overweight • Have high blood pressure • Have high cholesterol • Have advanced kidney disease • Drink too many alcoholic drinks • Smoke • Research also suggests that certain genes may make people more likely to develop diabetic neuropathy.
Causes	• Over time, high blood glucose levels, also called blood sugar, and high levels of fats, such as triglycerides, in the blood from diabetes can damage your nerves. • High blood glucose levels can also damage the small blood vessels that nourish your nerves with oxygen and nutrients. • Without enough oxygen and nutrients, your nerves cannot function well.

How Common is Diabetic Neuropathy?	• Although different types of diabetic neuropathy can affect people who have diabetes, research suggests that up to one-half of people with diabetes have peripheral neuropathy. More than 30 percent of people with diabetes have autonomic neuropathy. • The most common type of *focal neuropathy is carpal tunnel syndrome,* in which a nerve in your wrist is compressed. ○ Although less than 10 percent of people with diabetes feel symptoms of carpal tunnel syndrome, about 25 percent of people with diabetes have some nerve compression at the wrist.
Symptoms	• Your symptoms depend on which type of diabetic neuropathy you have. • In peripheral neuropathy, some people may have a loss of sensation in their feet, while others may have a burning or shooting pain in their lower legs. • Most nerve damage develops over many years, and some people may not notice symptoms of mild nerve damage for a long time. • In some people, severe pain begins suddenly.
What Problems does Diabetic Neuropathy Cause?	• *Peripheral neuropathy* can lead to foot complications, such as sores, ulcers, and infections, because nerve damage can make you lose feeling in your feet. As a result, you may not notice that your shoes are causing a sore or that you have injured your feet. • *Nerve damage* can also cause problems with balance and coordination, leading to falls and fractures. *(See Diabetes and Foot Problems)* ○ These problems may make it difficult for you to get around easily, causing you to lose some of your independence. • In some people with diabetes, nerve damage causes chronic pain, which can lead to anxiety and depression . • *Autonomic neuropathy* can cause problems with how your organs work, including problems with your heart rate and blood pressure, digestion, urination, and ability to sense when you have low blood glucose.
Prevention	To prevent diabetic neuropathy, it is important to manage your diabetes by managing your blood glucose, blood pressure, and cholesterol levels. You should also take the following steps to help prevent diabetes-related nerve damage: • Be physically active • Follow your diabetes meal plan • Get help to quit smoking • Limit alcoholic drinks to no more than one drink per day for women and no more than two drinks per day for men • Take any diabetes medicines and other medicines your doctor prescribes
How can I Prevent Diabetic Neuropathy from Getting Worse?	• If you have diabetic neuropathy, you should manage your diabetes, which means managing your blood glucose, blood pressure, cholesterol levels, and weight to keep nerve damage from getting worse. • Foot care is very important for all people with diabetes, and it's even more important if you have peripheral neuropathy. Check your feet for problems every day and take good care of your feet. • See your doctor for a neurological exam and a foot exam at least once a year—more often if you have foot problems. *(See Diabetes and Foot Problems)*

Peripheral Neuropathy

Peripheral neuropathy is a type of nerve damage that typically affects the feet and legs and sometimes affects the hands and arms. This type of neuropathy is very common. Up to one-half of people with diabetes have peripheral neuropathy.

PERIPHERAL NEUROPATHY
NERVE DAMAGE

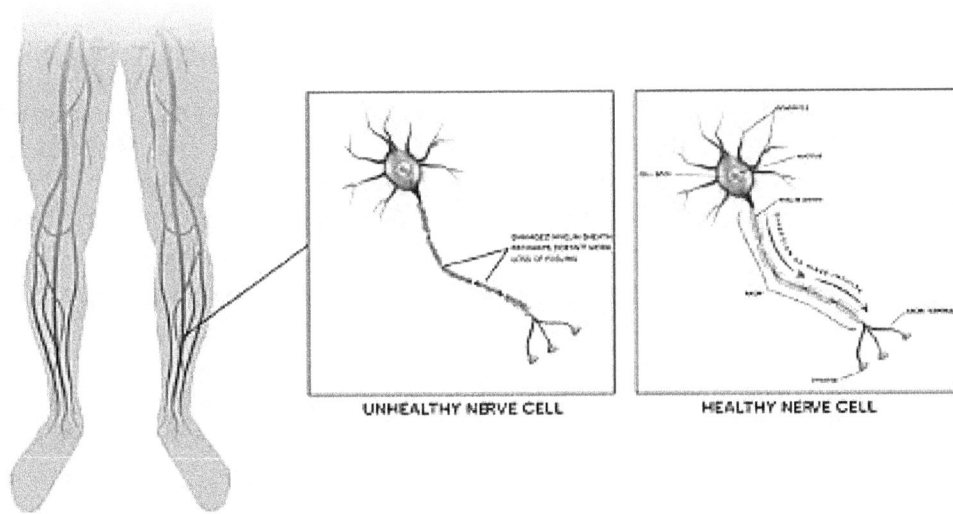

UNHEALTHY NERVE CELL   HEALTHY NERVE CELL

Causes	Over time, high blood glucose, also called blood sugar, and high levels of fats, such as triglycerides, in the blood from diabetes can damage your nerves and the small blood vessels that nourish your nerves, leading to peripheral neuropathy.
Symptoms	If you have peripheral neuropathy, your feet, legs, hands, or arms may feel: • Burning • Tingling, like "pins and needles" • Numb • Painful • Weak • You may feel extreme pain in your feet, legs, hands, and arms, even when they are touched lightly. You may also have problems sensing pain or temperature in these parts of your body. Symptoms are often worse at night. • Most of the time, you will have symptoms on both sides of your body. • However, you may have symptoms only on one side. *If you have peripheral neuropathy, you might experience:* • Changes in the way you walk • Loss of balance, which could make you fall more often • Loss of muscle tone in your hands and feet • Pain when you walk • Problems sensing movement or position • Swollen feet

What Problems does Peripheral Neuropathy Cause?	• Peripheral neuropathy can cause foot problems that lead to blisters and sores. If peripheral neuropathy causes you to lose feeling in your feet, you may not notice pressure or injuries that lead to blisters and sores. • Diabetes can make these wounds difficult to heal and increase the chance of infections. These sores and infections can lead to the loss of a toe, foot, or part of your leg. Finding and treating foot problems early can lower the chances that you will develop serious infections. • This type of diabetes-related nerve damage can also cause changes to the shape of your feet and toes. A rare condition that can occur in some people with diabetes is **Charcot's foot,** a problem in which the bones and tissue in your foot are damaged. • Peripheral neuropathy can make you more likely to lose your balance and fall, which can increase your chance of fractures and other injuries. • The chronic pain of peripheral neuropathy can also lead to grief, anxiety, and depression.
How can I Prevent the Problems Caused by Peripheral Neuropathy?	• You can prevent the problems caused by peripheral neuropathy by managing your diabetes, which means managing your blood glucose, blood pressure, and cholesterol. Staying close to your goal numbers can keep nerve damage from getting worse. • If you have diabetes, check your feet for problems every day and take good care of your feet. If you notice any foot problems, call or see your doctor right away. • Remove your socks and shoes in the exam room to remind your doctor to check your feet at every office visit. See your doctor for a foot exam at least once a year—more often if you have foot problems. Your doctor may send you to a podiatrist.

How do Doctors Treat Peripheral Neuropathy?	Doctors may prescribe medicine and other treatments for pain.
	
	Medicines for nerve pain
	Your doctor may prescribe medicines to help with pain, such as certain types of
	• Antidepressants, including
	  ○ Tricyclic antidepressants, such as nortriptyline , desipramine , imipramine , and amitriptyline
	  ○ Other types of antidepressants, such as duloxetine , venlafaxine , paroxetine , and citalopram
	• Anticonvulsants—medicines designed to treat seizures—such as gabapentin and pregabalin
	• Skin creams, patches, or sprays, such as lidocaine
	
	Although these medicines can help with the pain, they do not change the nerve damage. Therefore, if there is no improvement with a medicine to treat pain, there is no benefit to continuing to take it and another medication may be tried.
	• All medicines have side effects. Ask your doctor about the side effects of any medicines you take. Doctors don't recommend some medicines for older adults or for people with other health problems, such as heart disease.
	• Some doctors recommend avoiding over-the-counter pain medicines , such as acetaminophen and ibuprofen. These medicines may not work well for treating most nerve pain and can have side effects.
	
	Other treatments for nerve pain
	Your doctor may recommend other treatments for pain, including
	• Physical therapy to improve your strength and balance
	• A bed cradle, a device that keeps sheets and blankets off your legs and feet while you sleep
	• Diabetes experts have not made special recommendations about supplements for people with diabetes. For safety reasons, talk with your doctor before using supplements or any complementary or alternative medicines or medical practices.

Diabetes and Foot Problems

Foot problems are common in people with diabetes.
- You might be afraid you'll lose a toe, foot, or leg to diabetes, or know someone who has, but you can lower your chances of having diabetes-related foot problems by taking care of your feet every day.
- Managing your blood glucose levels, also called blood sugar, can also help keep your feet healthy

How can Diabetes Affect my Feet?	<ul><li>Over time, diabetes may cause nerve damage, also called diabetic neuropathy, that can cause tingling and pain and can make you lose feeling in your feet. When you lose feeling in your feet, you may not feel a pebble inside your sock or a blister on your foot, which can lead to cuts and sores. Cuts and sores can become infected.</li><li>Diabetes also can lower the amount of blood flow in your feet. Not having enough blood flowing to your legs and feet can make it hard for a sore or an infection to heal. Sometimes, a bad infection never heals. The infection might lead to gangrene.</li><li>Gangrene and foot ulcers that do not get better with treatment can lead to an amputation of your toe, foot, or part of your leg. A surgeon may perform an amputation to prevent a bad infection from spreading to the rest of your body, and to save your life. Good foot care is very important to prevent serious infections and gangrene.</li><li>Although rare, nerve damage from diabetes can lead to changes in the shape of your feet, such as Charcot's foot. Charcot's foot may start with redness, warmth, and swelling. Later, bones in your feet and toes can shift or break, which can cause your feet to have an odd shape, such as a "rocker bottom."</li></ul>
What can I do to Keep my Feet Healthy?	Work with your health care team to make a diabetes self-care plan, which is an action plan for how you will manage your diabetes. Your plan should include footcare. A foot doctor, also called a podiatrist, and other specialists may be part of your health care team. Include these steps in your footcare plan:<ul><li>Check your feet every day.</li><li>Wash your feet every day.</li><li>Smooth corns and calluses gently.</li><li>Trim your toenails straight across.</li><li>Wear shoes and socks at all times.</li><li>Protect your feet from hot and cold.</li><li>Keep the blood flowing to your feet.</li><li>Get a foot check at every health care visit.</li></ul> **Wash your feet every day**<ul><li>Wash your feet with soap in warm, not hot, water. Test the water to make sure it is not too hot. You can use a thermometer (90° to 95° F is safe) or your elbow to test the warmth of the water.</li><li>Do not soak your feet because your skin will get too dry.</li><li>After washing and drying your feet, put talcum powder or cornstarch between your toes.</li><li>Skin between the toes tends to stay moist. Powder will keep the skin dry to help prevent an infection.</li></ul>

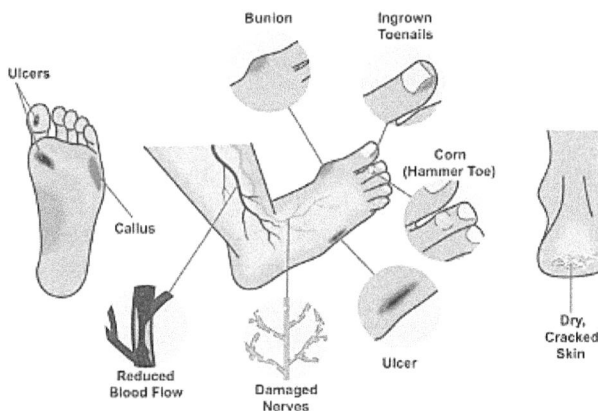

DIABETIC FOOT — Ulcers, Bunion, Ingrown Toenails, Corn (Hammer Toe), Callus, Reduced Blood Flow, Damaged Nerves, Ulcer, Dry, Cracked Skin

What can I do to Keep my Feet Healthy? *Continued*	**Check your feet every day** You may have foot problems but feel no pain in your feet. <ul><li>Checking your feet each day will help you spot problems early before they worsen.</li><li>A good way to remember is to check your feet each evening when you take off your shoes. Also check between your toes.</li><li>If you have trouble bending over to see your feet, try using a mirror to see them, or ask someone else to look at your feet.</li></ul>

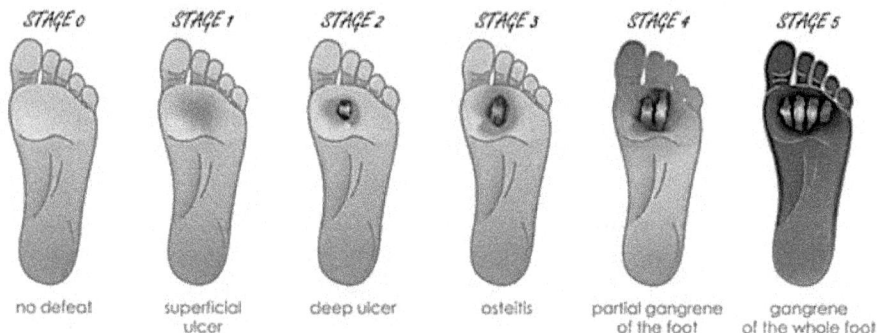

STAGE 0 — no defeat
STAGE 1 — superficial ulcer
STAGE 2 — deep ulcer
STAGE 3 — osteitis
STAGE 4 — partial gangrene of the foot
STAGE 5 — gangrene of the whole foot

Look for problems such as:
- Cuts, sores, or red spots
- Swelling or fluid-filled blisters
- Ingrown toenails, in which the edge of your nail grows into your skin
- Corns or calluses, which are spots of rough skin caused by too much rubbing or pressure on the same spot
- Plantar warts, which are flesh-colored growths on the bottom of the feet
- Athlete's foot
- Warm spots

If you have certain foot problems that make it more likely you will develop a sore on your foot, your doctor may recommend taking the temperature of the skin on different parts of your feet.
- A "hot spot" can be the first sign that a blister or an ulcer is starting.
- Cover a blister, cut, or sore with a bandage.
- Smooth corns and calluses as explained below.

Smooth corns and calluses gently
Thick patches of skin called corns or calluses can grow on the feet. If you have corns or calluses, talk with your foot doctor about the best way to care for these foot problems. If you have nerve damage, these patches can become ulcers.
- If your doctor tells you to, use a pumice stone to smooth corns and calluses after bathing or showering.
- A pumice stone is a type of rock used to smooth the skin. Rub gently, only in one direction, to avoid tearing the skin.

Do NOT:
- Cut corns and calluses
- Use corn plasters, which are medicated pads
- Use liquid corn and callus removers
- Cutting and over-the counter corn removal products can damage your skin and cause an infection.
  - To keep your skin smooth and soft, rub a thin coat of lotion, cream, or petroleum jelly on the tops and bottoms of your feet.
  - Do not put lotion or cream between your toes because moistness might cause an infection. |

What can I do to Keep my Feet Healthy? *Continued*	**Trim your toenails straight across** Trim your toenails, when needed, after you wash and dry your feet. <ul><li>Using toenail clippers, trim your toenails straight across.</li><li>Do not cut into the corners of your toenail.</li><li>Gently smooth each nail with an emery board or non-sharp nail file.</li><li>Trimming this way helps prevent cutting your skin and keeps the nails from growing into your skin.</li></ul> **Have a foot doctor trim your toenails if** <ul><li>You cannot see, feel, or reach your feet</li><li>Your toenails are thick or yellowed</li><li>Your nails curve and grow into the skin</li></ul> If you want to get a **pedicure at a salon**, you should bring your own nail tools to prevent getting an infection. <ul><li>You can ask your health care provider what other steps you can take to prevent infection.</li></ul> **Wear shoes and socks at all times.** <ul><li>Do not walk barefoot or in just socks – even when you are indoors. You could step on something and hurt your feet. You may not feel any pain and may not know that you hurt yourself.</li><li>Check the inside of your shoes before putting them on, to make sure the lining is smooth and free of pebbles or other objects.</li><li>Make sure you wear socks, stockings, or nylons with your shoes to keep from getting blisters and sores. Choose clean, lightly padded socks that fit well. Socks with no seams are best.</li></ul> Wear shoes that fit well and protect your feet. Here are some tips for finding the right type of shoes: <ul><li>Walking shoes and athletic shoes are good for daily wear. They support your feet and allow them to "breathe."</li><li>Do not wear vinyl or plastic shoes, because they do not stretch or "breathe."</li><li>When buying shoes, make sure they feel good and have enough room for your toes.</li><li>Buy shoes at the end of the day, when your feet are the largest, so that you can find the best fit.</li><li>If you have a bunion, or hammertoes, which are toes that curl under your feet, you may need extra-wide or deep shoes. Do not wear shoes with pointed toes or high heels, because they put too much pressure on your toes.</li><li>If your feet have changed shape, such as from *Charcot's* foot, you may need special shoes or shoe inserts, called orthotics.<ul><li>You also may need inserts if you have bunions, hammertoes, or other foot problems.</li></ul></li><li>When breaking in new shoes, only wear them for a few hours at first and then check your feet for areas of soreness.</li></ul> Medicare Part B insurance and other health insurance programs may help pay for these special shoes or inserts. Ask your insurance plan if it covers your special shoes or inserts.

What can I do to Keep my Feet Healthy? *Continued*	**Protect your feet from hot and cold** If you have nerve damage from diabetes, you may burn your feet and not know you did. Take the following steps to protect your feet from heat: <ul><li>Wear shoes at the beach and on hot pavement.</li><li>Put sunscreen on the tops of your feet to prevent sunburn.</li><li>Keep your feet away from heaters and open fires.</li><li>Do not put a hot water bottle or heating pad on your feet.</li><li>Wear socks in bed if your feet get cold. In the winter, wear lined, waterproof boots to keep your feet warm and dry.</li></ul> **Keep the blood flowing to your feet** Try the following tips to improve blood flow to your feet: <ul><li>Put your feet up when you are sitting.</li><li>Wiggle your toes for a few minutes throughout the day. Move your ankles up and down and in and out to help blood flow in your feet and legs.</li><li>Do not wear tight socks or elastic stockings. Do not try to hold up loose socks with rubber bands.</li><li>Be more physically active. Choose activities that are easy on your feet, such as walking, dancing, yoga or stretching, swimming, or bike riding.</li><li>Stop smoking.</li></ul> **Get a foot check at every health care visit** Ask your health care team to check your feet at each visit. Take off your shoes and socks when you're in the exam room so they will remember to check your feet. At least once a year, get a thorough foot exam, including a check of the feeling and pulses in your feet. Get a thorough foot exam at each health care visit if you have: <ul><li>Changes in the shape of your feet</li><li>Loss of feeling in your feet</li><li>Peripheral artery disease</li><li>Had foot ulcers or an amputation in the past</li></ul> 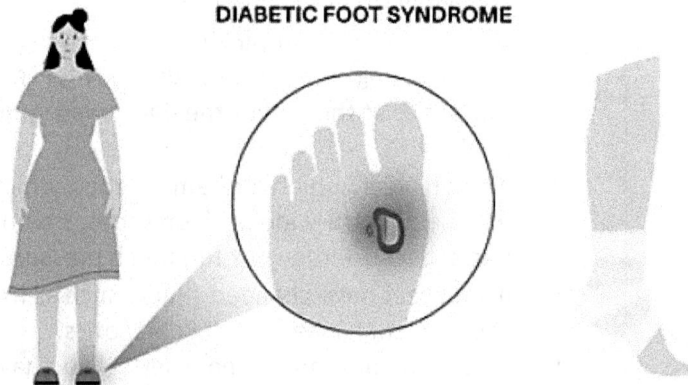 DIABETIC FOOT SYNDROME
When should I see my health care provider about foot problems?	Call your health care provider right away if you have: <ul><li>A cut, blister, or bruise on your foot that does not start to heal after a few days</li><li>Skin on your foot that becomes red, warm, or painful—signs of a possible infection</li><li>A callus with dried blood inside of it, which often can be the first sign of a wound under the callus</li><li>A foot infection that becomes black and smelly—signs you might have gangrene</li></ul> Ask your provider to refer you to a foot doctor, or podiatrist, if needed.

Hypoglycemia

Hypoglycemia, also called low blood glucose or low blood sugar, occurs when the level of glucose in your blood drops below normal.

- For many people with diabetes, that means a level of 70 milligrams per deciliter (mg/dL) or less.
- Your numbers might be different, so check with your health care provider to find out what level is too low for you.

Symptoms	• Symptoms of hypoglycemia tend to come on quickly and can vary from person to person. You may have one or more mild-to-moderate symptoms listed in the table below. Sometimes people don't feel any symptoms. • Severe hypoglycemia is when your blood glucose level becomes so low that you're unable to treat yourself and need help from another person. Severe hypoglycemia is dangerous and needs to be treated right away. This condition is more common in people with type 1 diabetes.

Hypoglycemia Symptoms		
Mild-to-Moderate		**Severe**
• Shaky or jittery • Sweaty • Hungry • Headachy • Blurred vision • Sleepy or tired • Dizzy or lightheaded • Confused or disoriented • Pale	• Uncoordinated • Irritable or nervous • Argumentative or combative • Changed behavior or personality • Trouble concentrating • Weak • Fast or irregular heart beat	• Unable to eat or drink • Seizures or convulsions (jerky movements) • Unconsciousness

HYPOGLYCEMIA

Dizziness   Sweating   Mood swings   Trembling   Hunger

Blurred vision   Tachycardia   Pallor   Headache   Fatigue

Some symptoms of hypoglycemia during sleep are:
- Crying out or having nightmares
- Sweating enough to make your pajamas or sheets damp
- Feeling tired, irritable, or confused after waking up

Causes	• Hypoglycemia can be a side effect of insulin or other types of diabetes medicines that help your body make more insulin. • Two types of diabetes pills can cause hypoglycemia: sulfonylureas and meglitinides. Ask your health care team if your diabetes medicine can cause hypoglycemia. • Although other diabetes medicines don't cause hypoglycemia by themselves, they can increase the chances of hypoglycemia if you also take insulin, a sulfonylurea, or a meglitinide.

What other Factors Contribute to Hypoglycemia in Diabetes?	If you take insulin or diabetes medicines that increase the amount of insulin your body makes—but don't match your medications with your food or physical activity—you could develop hypoglycemia. The following factors can make hypoglycemia more likely: • Not eating enough carbohydrates (carbs): When you eat foods containing carbohydrates, your digestive system breaks down the sugars and starches into glucose. Glucose then enters your bloodstream and raises your blood glucose level. If you don't eat enough carbohydrates to match your medication, your blood glucose could drop too low. • Skipping or delaying a meal. If you skip or delay a meal, your blood glucose could drop too low. Hypoglycemia also can occur when you are asleep and haven't eaten for several hours. • Increasing physical activity. Increasing your physical activity level beyond your normal routine can lower your blood glucose level for up to 24 hours after the activity. • Drinking too much alcohol without enough food • Alcohol makes it harder for your body to keep your blood glucose level steady, especially if you haven't eaten in a while. The effects of alcohol can also keep you from feeling the symptoms of hypoglycemia, which may lead to severe hypoglycemia. • Being sick. When you're sick, you may not be able to eat as much or keep food down, which can cause low blood glucose.
Prevention	If you are taking insulin, a sulfonylurea, or a meglitinide, using your diabetes management plan and working with your health care team to adjust your plan as needed can help you prevent hypoglycemia. The following actions can also help prevent hypoglycemia: ***Check blood glucose levels*** Knowing your blood glucose level can help you decide how much medicine to take, what food to eat, and how physically active to be. To find out your blood glucose level, check yourself with a blood glucose meter as often as your doctor advises. • *Hypoglycemia unawareness.* Sometimes people with diabetes don't feel or recognize the symptoms of hypoglycemia, a problem called hypoglycemia unawareness. If you have had hypoglycemia without feeling any symptoms, you may need to check your blood glucose more often so you know when you need to treat your hypoglycemia or take steps to prevent it. Be sure to check your blood glucose before you drive. • If you have hypoglycemia unawareness or have hypoglycemia often, ask your health care provider about a continuous glucose monitor (CGM). A CGM checks your blood glucose level at regular times throughout the day and night. CGMs can tell you if your blood glucose is falling quickly and sound an alarm if your blood glucose falls too low. CGM alarms can wake you up if you have hypoglycemia during sleep. ***Eat regular meals and snacks*** • Your meal plan is key to preventing hypoglycemia. Eat regular meals and snacks with the correct amount of carbohydrates to help keep your blood glucose level from going too low. Also, if you drink alcoholic beverages, it's best to eat some food at the same time. ***Be physically active safely*** • Physical activity can lower your blood glucose during the activity and for hours afterward. To help prevent hypoglycemia, you may need to check your blood glucose before, during, and after physical activity and adjust your medicine or carbohydrate intake. For example, you might eat a snack before being physically active or decrease your insulin dose as directed by your health care provider to keep your blood glucose from dropping too low. • Tell your health care team if you have had hypoglycemia. Your health care team may adjust your diabetes medicines or other aspects of your management plan. Learn about balancing your medicines, eating plan, and physical activity to prevent hypoglycemia. • Ask if you should have a glucagon emergency kit to carry with you at all times.

How do I Treat Hypoglycemia	• If you begin to feel one or more hypoglycemia symptoms, check your blood glucose. If your blood glucose level is below your target or less than 70, eat or drink 15 grams of carbohydrates right away. Examples include:
	  ○ Four glucose tablets or one tube of glucose gel
	  ○ 1/2 cup (4 ounces) of fruit juice—not low-calorie or reduced sugar*
	  ○ 1/2 can (4 to 6 ounces) of soda—not low-calorie or reduced sugar
	  ○ 1 tablespoon of sugar, honey, or corn syrup
	  ○ 2 tablespoons of raisins
	• Wait 15 minutes and check your blood glucose again. If your glucose level is still low, eat or drink another 15 grams of glucose or carbohydrates. Check your blood glucose again after another 15 minutes. Repeat these steps until your glucose level is back to normal.
	• If your next meal is more than 1 hour away, have a snack to keep your blood glucose level in your target range. Try crackers or a piece of fruit.
	
	People who have kidney disease should NOT drink orange juice for their 15 grams of carbohydrates because it contains a lot of potassium.
	Apple, grape, or cranberry juice are good options.
	
	Treating hypoglycemia if you take acarbose or miglitol
	• If you take acarbose or miglitol along with diabetes medicines that can cause hypoglycemia, you will need to take glucose tablets or glucose gel if your blood glucose level is too low.
	• Eating or drinking other sources of carbohydrates won't raise your blood glucose level quickly enough.

What if I have Severe Hypoglycemia and Can't Treat Myself?	• Someone will need to give you a glucagon injection if you have severe hypoglycemia. An injection of glucagon will quickly raise your blood glucose level. ○ Talk with your health care provider about when and how to use a glucagon emergency kit. If you have an emergency kit, check the date on the package to make sure it hasn't expired. • If you are likely to have severe hypoglycemia, teach your family, friends, and coworkers when and how to give you a glucagon injection. Also, tell your family, friends, and coworkers to call 911 right away after giving you a glucagon injection or if you don't have a glucagon emergency kit with you. • If you have hypoglycemia often or have had severe hypoglycemia, you should wear a medical alert bracelet or pendant. A medical alert ID tells other people that you have diabetes and need care right away. • Getting prompt care can help prevent the serious problems that hypoglycemia can cause.

Physical Activity

Physical Activity	- Lowers blood glucose levels - Lowers blood pressure - Improves blood flow - Burns extra calories so you can keep your weight down if needed - Improves your mood - Can prevent falls and improve memory in older adults - May help you sleep better 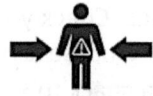 VISCERAL OBESITY　　HYPERTENSION　　INSULIN RESISTANCE　　HIGH TRIGLYCERIDES　　LOW HDL-CHOLESTEROL If you are overweight, combining physical activity with a reduced-calorie eating plan can lead to even more benefits. - In the Look AHEAD: Action for Health in Diabetes study, overweight adults with type 2 diabetes who ate less and moved more had greater long-term health benefits compared to those who didn't make these changes. These benefits included improved cholesterol levels, less sleep apnea, and being able to move around more easily. - Even small amounts of physical activity can help. Experts suggest that you aim for at least 30 minutes of moderate or vigorous physical activity 5 days of the week. - Moderate activity feels somewhat hard, and vigorous activity is intense and feels hard. If you want to lose weight or maintain weight loss, you may need to do 60 minutes or more of physical activity 5 days of the week. - Be patient. It may take a few weeks of physical activity before you see changes in your health.
How can I be Physically Active Safely if I have Diabetes?	Be sure to drink water before, during, and after exercise to stay well hydrated. The following are some other tips for safe physical activity when you have diabetes. *Plan ahead* - Talk with your health care team before you start a new physical activity routine, especially if you have other health problems. Your health care team will tell you a target range for your blood glucose level and suggest how you can be active safely. - Your health care team also can help you decide the best time of day for you to do physical activity based on your daily schedule, meal plan, and diabetes medicines. - If you take insulin, you need to balance the activity that you do with your insulin doses and meals so you don't get low blood glucose. *Preventing low blood glucose* - Because physical activity lowers your blood glucose, you should protect yourself against low blood glucose levels, also called hypoglycemia. You are most likely to have hypoglycemia if you take insulin or certain other diabetes medicines, such as a sulfonylurea. - Hypoglycemia also can occur after a long intense workout or if you have skipped a meal before being active. Hypoglycemia can happen during or up to 24 hours after physical activity. - Planning is key to preventing hypoglycemia. For instance, if you take insulin, your health care provider might suggest you take less insulin or eat a small snack with carbohydrates before, during, or after physical activity, especially intense activity. - You may need to check your blood glucose level before, during, and right after you are physically active.

How can I Be Physically Active Safely if I have Diabetes? *Continued*	***Stay safe when blood glucose is high - Type 1 Diabetes*** • If you have *type 1* diabetes, *avoid* vigorous physical activity when you have ketones in your blood or urine. o Ketones are chemicals your body might make when your blood glucose level is too high, a condition called hyperglycemia, and your insulin level is too low. • If you are physically active when you have ketones in your blood or urine, your blood glucose level may go even higher. Ask your health care team what level of ketones are dangerous for you and how to test for them. • Ketones are uncommon in people with type 2 diabetes. ***Take care of your feet*** • People with diabetes may have problems with their feet because of poor blood flow and nerve damage that can result from high blood glucose levels. • To help prevent foot problems, you should wear comfortable, supportive shoes and take care of your feet before, during, and after physical activity.
What Physical Activities should I do?	Most kinds of physical activity can help you take care of your diabetes. • Certain activities may be unsafe for some people, such as those with low vision or nerve damage to their feet. • Ask your health care team what physical activities are safe for you. Many people choose walking with friends or family members for their activity. • Doing different types of physical activity each week will give you the most health benefits. Mixing it up also helps reduce boredom and lower your chance of getting hurt. **Try these options for physical activity.** ***Add extra activity to your daily routine*** If you have been inactive or you are trying a new activity, start slowly, with 5 to 10 minutes a day. Then add a little more time each week. Increase daily activity by spending less time in front of a TV or other screen. Try these simple ways to add physical activities in your life each day: • Walk around while you talk on the phone or during TV commercials. • Do chores, such as work in the garden, rake leaves, clean the house, or wash the car. • Park at the far end of the shopping center parking lot and walk to the store. • Take the stairs instead of the elevator. • Make your family outings active, such as a family bike ride or a walk in a park. If you are sitting for a long time, such as working at a desk or watching TV, do some light activity for 3 minutes or more every half hour. Light activities include: • Leg lifts or extensions • Overhead arm stretches • Desk chair swivels • Torso twists • Side lunges • Walking/marching in place

What Physical Activities should I do?
 	
Continued
	Do aerobic exercise
	Aerobic exercise is activity that makes your heart beat faster and makes you breathe harder. You should aim for doing aerobic exercise for 30 minutes a day most days of the week. You do not have to do all the activity at one time. You can split up these minutes into a few times throughout the day.
	
	To get the most out of your activity, exercise at a moderate to vigorous level, try:
	• Walking briskly or hiking
	• Climbing stairs
	• Swimming or a water-aerobics class
	• Dancing
	• Riding a bicycle or a stationary bicycle
	• Taking an exercise class
	• Playing basketball, tennis, or other sports
	
	Talk with your health care team about how to warm up and cool down before and after you exercise.
	
	Do strength training to build muscle
	• Strength training is a light or moderate physical activity that builds muscle and helps keep your bones healthy. Strength training is important for both men and women.
	• When you have more muscle and less body fat, you'll burn more calories. Burning more calories can help you lose and keep off extra weight.
	• You can do strength training with hand weights, elastic bands, or weight machines. Try to do strength training two to three times a week.
	• Start with a light weight. Slowly increase the size of your weights as your muscles become stronger.
	
	Do stretching exercises
	• Stretching exercises are light or moderate physical activity. When you stretch, you increase your flexibility, lower your stress, and help prevent sore muscles.
	• You can choose from many types of stretching exercises.
	• Yoga is a type of stretching that focuses on your breathing and helps you relax. Even if you have problems moving or balancing, certain types of yoga can help.
	  o For instance, chair yoga has stretches you can do when sitting in a chair or holding onto a chair while standing.
	  o Your health care team can suggest whether yoga is right for you.
	
	Refer to the 2nd section on Home Exercise for more information about exercises:
	• Warm up/Cool Down
	• Flexibility/Stretching
	• Core/Abdominal
	• Balance
	• Strengthening
	• Lower Extremity Strengthening in lying or seated
	• Upper Extremity Strengthening
	• Agility
	• Aerobics / Endurance

Special Considerations for People with Diabetes *CDC – Diabetes – Get Active*	It is important to understand the correlation between blood sugar and exercise. Before starting any physical activity, check with your health care provider to talk about the best physical activities for you. Be sure to discuss which activities you like, how to prepare, and what you should avoid. <ul><li>Drink plenty of fluids while being physically active to prevent dehydration (harmful loss of water in the body).</li><li>Make sure to check your blood sugar before being physically active, especially if you take insulin.</li><li>If it's **below 100 mg/dL,** you may need to eat a small snack containing 15-30 grams of carbohydrates, such as 2 tablespoons of raisins or ½ cup of fruit juice or regular soda (not diet), or glucose tablets so your blood sugar doesn't fall too low while being physically active.<ul><li>Low blood sugar (hypoglycemia) can be very serious.</li></ul></li><li>If it's **above 240 mg/dL**, your blood sugar may be too high (hyperglycemia) to be active safely.<ul><li>Test your urine for ketones – substances made when your body breaks down fat for energy. The presence of ketones indicates that your body doesn't have enough insulin to control your blood sugar.</li><li>If you are physically active when you have high ketone levels, you risk ketoacidosis – a serious diabetes complication that needs immediate treatment.</li></ul></li><li>When you're physically active, wear cotton socks and athletic shoes that fit well and are comfortable.</li><li>After your activity, check to see how it has affected your blood glucose level.</li><li>After being physically active, check your feet for sores, blisters, irritation, cuts, or other injuries.</li><li>*Call your health care provider if an injury doesn't begin to heal after 2 days.*</li></ul> *CDC – Diabetes – Get Active*

Diet

What Foods can I Eat?	You may worry that having diabetes means going without foods you enjoy.
	• The good news is that you can still eat your favorite foods, but you might need to eat smaller portions or enjoy them less often.
	• Your health care team will help create a diabetes meal plan for you that meets your needs and likes.
	• The key to eating with diabetes is to eat a variety of healthy foods from all food groups, in the amounts your meal plan outlines.
	
	The food groups are:
	• Vegetables
	    ○ Non-starchy: includes broccoli, carrots, greens, peppers, and tomatoes
	    ○ Starchy: includes potatoes, corn, and green peas
	• Fruits—includes oranges, melon, berries, apples, bananas, and grapes
	• Grains—at least half of your grains for the day should be whole grains
	    ○ Includes wheat, rice, oats, cornmeal, barley, and quinoa
	    ○ Examples: bread, pasta, cereal, and tortillas
	• Protein
	    ○ Lean meat
	    ○ Chicken or turkey without the skin
	    ○ Fish
	    ○ Eggs
	    ○ Nuts and peanuts
	    ○ Dried beans and certain peas, such as chickpeas and split peas
	    ○ Meat substitutes, such as tofu
	• Dairy—nonfat or low fat
	    ○ Milk or lactose-free milk if you have lactose intolerance
	    ○ Yogurt
	    ○ Cheese
	
	Learn more about the food groups at the U.S. Department of Agriculture's (USDA) *ChooseMyPlate.gov.*
	
	Eat foods with heart-healthy fats, which mainly come from these foods:
	• Oils that are liquid at room temperature, such as canola and olive oil
	• Nuts and seeds
	• Heart-healthy fish such as salmon, tuna, and mackerel
	• Avocado
	• Use oils when cooking food instead of butter, cream, shortening, lard, or stick margarine.

What Foods and Drinks should I Limit?	Foods and drinks to limit include
	• Fried foods and other foods high in saturated fat and trans fat
	• Foods high in salt, also called sodium
	• Sweets, such as baked goods, candy, and ice cream
	• Beverages with added sugars, such as juice, regular soda, and regular sports or energy drinks
	• Drink water instead of sweetened beverages. Consider using a sugar substitute in your coffee or tea.
	• If you drink alcohol, drink moderately—no more than one drink a day if you're a woman or two drinks a day if you're a man.
	    ○ If you use insulin or diabetes medicines that increase the amount of insulin your body makes, alcohol can make your blood glucose level drop too low. This is especially true if you haven't eaten in a while.
	    ○ It's best to eat some food when you drink alcohol.

Diet	Diabetes
When should I Eat?	Some people with diabetes need to eat at about the same time each day. Others can be more flexible with the timing of their meals. • Depending on your diabetes medicines or type of insulin, you may need to eat the same amount of carbohydrates at the same time each day. If you take "mealtime" insulin, your eating schedule can be more flexible. • If you use certain diabetes medicines or insulin and you skip or delay a meal, your blood glucose level can drop too low. • Ask your health care team when you should eat and whether you should eat before and after physical activity.
How Much can I Eat?	Eating the right amount of food will also help you manage your blood glucose level and your weight. • Your health care team can help you figure out how much food and how many calories you should eat each day.
Weight-loss Planning	If you are overweight or have obesity, work with your health care team to create a weight-loss plan. • The Body Weight Planner can help you tailor your calorie and physical activity plans to reach and maintain your goal weight. • To lose weight, you need to eat fewer calories and replace less healthy foods with foods lower in calories, fat, and sugar. • If you have diabetes, are overweight or obese, and are planning to have a baby, you should try to lose any excess weight before you become pregnant. ○ Learn more about planning for pregnancy if you have diabetes.
Meal Plan Methods	Two common ways to help you plan how much to eat if you have diabetes are the plate method and carbohydrate counting, also called carb counting. Check with your health care team about the method that's best for you. *Plate method* • The plate method helps you control your portion sizes. You don't need to count calories. The plate method shows the amount of each food group you should eat. This method works best for lunch and dinner. • Use a 9-inch plate. Put non-starchy vegetables on half of the plate; a meat or other protein on one-fourth of the plate; and a grain or other starch on the last one-fourth. • Starches include starchy vegetables such as corn and peas. You also may eat a small bowl of fruit or a piece of fruit and drink a small glass of milk as included in your meal plan. You can find many different combinations of food and more details about using the plate method from the American Diabetes Association's Create Your Plate. • Your daily eating plan also may include small snacks between meals. *Portion sizes* You can use everyday objects or your hand to judge the size of a portion. • 1 serving of meat or poultry is the palm of your hand or a deck of cards • 1 3-ounce serving of fish is a checkbook • 1 serving of cheese is six dice • 1/2 cup of cooked rice or pasta is a rounded handful or a tennis ball • 1 serving of a pancake or waffle is a DVD • 2 tablespoons of peanut butter is a ping-pong ball

Meal Plan Methods *Continued*	***Carbohydrate counting*** Carbohydrate counting involves keeping track of the amount of carbohydrates you eat and drink each day. <ul><li>Because carbohydrates turn into glucose in your body, they affect your blood glucose level more than other foods do.</li><li>Carb counting can help you manage your blood glucose level.</li><li>If you take insulin, counting carbohydrates can help you know how much insulin to take.</li><li>Carbohydrate counting is a meal planning tool for people with diabetes who take insulin, but not all people with diabetes need to count carbohydrates.<ul><li>Your health care team can help you create a personal eating plan that will best meet your needs.</li></ul></li></ul>The amount of carbohydrates in foods is measured in grams. To count carbohydrate grams in what you eat, you'll need to: <ul><li>Learn which foods have carbohydrates</li><li>Read the Nutrition Facts food label or learn to estimate the number of grams of carbohydrate in the foods you eat.</li><li>Add the grams of carbohydrate from each food you eat to get your total for each meal and for the day.</li></ul>Most carbohydrates come from starches, fruits, milk, and sweets. <ul><li>Try to limit carbohydrates with added sugars or those with refined grains, such as white bread and white rice.</li><li>Instead, eat carbohydrates from fruit, vegetables, whole grains, beans, and low-fat or non-fat milk.</li></ul>
What is Medical Nutrition Therapy?	<ul><li>Medical nutrition therapy is a service provided by a Registered Dietician to create personal eating plans based on your needs and likes.</li><li>For people with diabetes, medical nutrition therapy has been shown to improve diabetes management.</li><li>Medicare pays for medical nutrition therapy for people with diabetes. If you have insurance other than Medicare, ask if it covers medical nutrition therapy for diabetes.</li></ul>
Will Supplements and Vitamins Help my Diabetes?	<ul><li>No clear proof exists that taking dietary supplements such as vitamins, minerals, herbs, or spices can help manage diabetes.</li><li>You may need supplements if you cannot get enough vitamins and minerals from foods.</li><li>Talk with your health care provider before you take any dietary supplement since some can cause side effects or affect how your medicines work.</li></ul>

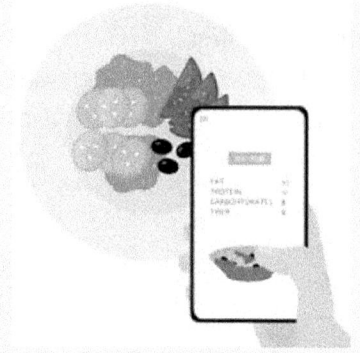

Diabetes References

NIH – National Institute of Diabetes and Digestive and Kidney Diseases:

Diabetes and Foot Problems - https://www.niddk.nih.gov/health-information/diabetes/overview/preventing-problems/foot-problems

Diabetes Diet, Eating, & Physical Activity - https://www.niddk.nih.gov/health-information/diabetes/overview/diet-eating-physical-activity

Diabetes Overview - https://www.niddk.nih.gov/health-information/diabetes/overview

Diabetic Neuropathy - https://www.niddk.nih.gov/health-information/diabetes/overview/preventing-problems/nerve-damage-diabetic-neuropathies

Gestational Diabetes - https://www.niddk.nih.gov/health-information/diabetes/overview/what-is-diabetes/gestational

Insulin Resistance - https://www.niddk.nih.gov/health-information/diabetes/overview/what-is-diabetes/prediabetes-insulin-resistance

Insulin, Medicines, & Other Diabetes Treatments - https://www.niddk.nih.gov/health-information/diabetes/overview/insulin-medicines-treatments

Low Blood Glucose (Hypoglycemia) - https://www.niddk.nih.gov/health-information/diabetes/overview/preventing-problems/low-blood-glucose-hypoglycemia

Peripheral Neuropathy - https://www.niddk.nih.gov/health-information/diabetes/overview/preventing-problems/nerve-damage-diabetic-neuropathies/peripheral-neuropathy

Type 1 Diabetes - https://www.niddk.nih.gov/health-information/diabetes/overview/what-is-diabetes/type-1-diabetes

Type 2 Diabetes - https://www.niddk.nih.gov/health-information/diabetes/overview/what-is-diabetes/type-2-diabetes

Other References

Cleveland Clinic https://my.clevelandclinic.org/health/diseases/21147-hyperosmolar-hyperglycemic-state

Diabetes – *Get Active* – CDC https://www.cdc.gov/diabetes/managing/active.html

MedLine Plus - *Diabetic ketoacidosis* - https://medlineplus.gov/ency/article/000320.htm

WebMD - *What are Ketones?* - https://www.webmd.com/diabetes/qa/what-are-ketones

Quick Summary this Section

Safety First

- Benefits / Before Starting a Routine
- Averages, Body Temperature
- Respiration, Blood Pressure, Heart Rate
- How to Monitor Intensity of Heart Rate
- Temperature – Heat and Cold
- Dehydration; Altitude

Components of a Conditioning Program

- Warm up/cool down
- Duration, Frequency, Intensity & Movement Patterns
- Breathing – Diaphragmatic, Pursed lip and with Exercise
- Anatomy
- Equipment That May be Needed

Self-Tests:

- Prior to starting program

Exercise Worksheets:

- Exercises below with:
  - Exercise name and number for section
    - Reps, Sets, How many times a day and how long a stretch should be held (Ex. 20 seconds)

EXERCISE Flexibility (Stretching)	EXERCISE NUMBER	PAGE	REPS	SETS	X DAY	HOLD
PRAYER STRETCH and LATERAL	53					

Exercises:

- Myofascial release
- Flexibility / Stretches / ROM
- Core / Abdominal
- Strengthening - Upper and Lower Extremity
- Balance > Lower Extremity Standing Exercises
- Agility
- Endurance/Aerobic Capacity
- Calories
- Worksheet with room for notes under each section

EXERCISE Core / Stability / Balance	EXERCISE NUMBER	NOTES
PRONE BALL	27	

References

PHYSICAL AND PSYCHOLOGICAL BENEFITS OF KEEPING PHYSICALLY FIT

- Contributes positively to maintaining a healthy weight, building and maintaining healthy bone density, muscle strength, joint mobility, reducing surgical risks, and strengthening the immune system.
- Helps to prevent or treat serious and life-threatening chronic conditions such as high blood pressure, obesity, heart disease, Type 2 diabetes, insomnia, and depression.
- Endurance exercise before meals lowers blood glucose more than the same exercise after meals.
- It also improves mental health, helps prevent depression, helps to promote or maintain positive self-esteem, and can even augment an individual's sex appeal or body image.

(Physical Exercise - Wikipedia)

Before starting a routine here are some factors to consider

AGE	Men over 45 and women over 55 should have medical evaluation before starting a vigorous exercise program. If you will be participating in low to moderate exercise, it is suggested that those with, or have signs and symptoms of cardiopulmonary disease, set up a medical evaluation.
MEDICAL AND PHYSICAL CONDITION	It is very important for you to be aware of any medical or physical problems that may impede your performance. **If you have any of the following issues, please see a medical doctor and/or physical therapist to address issues before starting an exercise program:** • Cardiac issues • Pulmonary issues • Arthritis • Joint pain • Back pain • Diabetes • Acute or Chronic issues, such as, but not limited to, Parkinson's, Stroke, Autoimmune Diseases, Metabolic Disease or Orthopedic disorders/joint replacements.

VITAL SIGN AVERAGES

Adult (resting)

Body Temperature	98.6 Fahrenheit under tongue.
Respiration	12-20 breaths per minute

Blood Pressure
 	
Systolic/Diastolic
	120/80.
	Systolic is when the heart pumps blood to the body / Diastolic is blood that remains in arteries when the heart relaxes.
	Pre-hypertension: 120-139/80-89.
	Hypertension:
	  Stage I 140-159/90-99
	  Stage II over 160/100

Resting pulse	**Men:** 70 beats per minute. **Women:** 75 beats per minute.

HOW to MONITOR EXERCISE INTENSITY

Ways to monitor heart rate (HR):

Talk Test Method	This is a simple, subjective method for the beginner to determine your comfort zone while exercising. Are you able to breathe and talk comfortably throughout the workout without gasping for air? If not, reduce your activity level, catch your breath, and resume at a slower pace.
Heart Rate monitor or Watch	This is a device you wear on your wrist or chest, which allows you to measure your heart rate in real time. These devices range in price at about $50.00 for just a basic HR monitor or higher with other bells and whistles. Some of the popular manufacturers are Fitbit, Apple Watch, Garmin and Samsung Galaxy among others. (See *Target Heart Rate*)
Rate of Perceived Exertion	This method was designed by Dr. Gunnar Borg and is often called the Borg Scale (revised). It rates what you feel your level of exertion is from a scale of 1-10, one being at rest and ten at maximal exertion. A rate of 5-7 is recommended, somewhere between somewhat hard and very hard. Like the talk test method, this is subjective and should be used with HR monitoring.
Training Heart Rate	Measuring Heart Rate: Place your first and second finger over the pulse site and gently apply pressure. Palpate the number of beats for a full minute or 30 sec x 2, 15 sec x 4 or 6 sec x 10. If you have in irregular heartbeat, it is suggested counting the full 60 seconds. Do not use the thumb, as this has its own pulse.
	Take your pulse after you've been exercising for at least five minutes. An easy way to check your pulse without interrupting your workout too much is to take a quick 6-second count and then multiply that number by 10 to get your heart rate in beats per minute (BPM). Make sure your pulse is within your target heart rate zone (*see below*). You can then increase or decrease your intensity based on your heart rate. You can also wear a heart rate monitor. Radial: Wrist following line from base of thumb. Carotid: Side of larynx.
Target heart rate range (THR)	**Beginner or low fitness level**: 50-60% **Intermediate or average fitness level:** 60-70% **Advanced or high fitness level:** 75-85%
Percent of maximal heart rate	220 - Age = predicted maximum heart rate (HR). To get the desired exercise intensity, multiply the predicted maximal HR by the percentage. For example, a woman who is 40 years old of Intermediate fitness level would use the following equation at a 70% target heart rate: 220 – 40 (age) =180 predicted maximal HR. 180 x 0.70 (THR) = 126 BPM - desired exercise HR.
Karvonen Formula	Percentage of Heart-rate reserve. This formula factors in the resting HR as well, which will make the target heart rate higher than just the percentage of maximal heart rate. To figure this out, take the predicted maximal heart rate as above with a resting HR prior to exercise. Maximal HR – resting heart rate (RHR) = heart rate reserve; multiply by intensity + RHR + Target HR. See example under Percentage of maximal HR. Rest heart rate = 80. 220 – 40 (age) =180 (as above) – 80 (RHR) = 100 x 0.70 (THR) = 70 + 80 = 150 Target HR.

TEMPERATURE – HEAT and COLD

HEAT

Avoid exercise in the hottest part of the day, as well as in humid weather. People need to sweat to regulate internal body temperature and must evaporate to dissipate heat. During hot, humid weather, sweat cannot evaporate, and therefore cannot cool the body down. It is also important to drink plenty of cool water during exercise, about 7-10 oz. every 10-20 minutes during exercise (see *Dehydration*).

Heat cramps:	• Severe cramps that begin in hands, feet or calves • Hard, tense muscles
Heat exhaustion: Requires immediate medical attention, although not usually life threatening	• Fatigue • Nausea • Headache • Excessive thirst • Muscle aches and cramps • Confusion or anxiety • Weakness • Severe sweats that can be accompanied by cold, clammy skin • Slow heartbeat (decreased pulse rate) • Dizziness or fainting • Agitation
Heat Stroke: Can occur suddenly, with or without warning from heat exhaustion. Obtain immediate medical attention, as this can be *fatal*	• Nausea and vomiting • Headache • Increased body temperature, but DECREASED sweating. • Hot, flushed, DRY skin • Dizziness • Fatigue • Rapid heart rate • Shortness of breath • Decreased urination or may have blood in the urine. • Confusion or loss of consciousness • Convulsions

COLD

It is just as important to drink plenty of water when exercising in the cold weather secondary to increased urine production.   Be sure to dress in layers to help self-regulate body temperature. This simply involves taking off or putting back on clothing as dictated by the changing weather conditions. Choose clothing that will keep moisture out and away from the skin, such as Gortex® brand. Clothing that stays wet because of sweat will decrease your body temperature.

Hypothermia-Mild: A body temperature that is below normal. People with hypothermia are usually not aware of their condition due to confusion or being overly focused on their current activity. Hypothermia may or may not include shivering in the early stages	• Confusion • Lack of coordination • Fatigue • Nausea or vomiting • Dizziness
Hypothermia	• Shivering • Slurred speech • Mumbling • Clumsiness • Difficulty speaking • Stumbling • Poor decision making • Drowsiness • Weak pulse • Shallow breathing • Progressive loss of consciousness

DEHYDRATION

Excessive loss of body fluid (which can include water and solutes, usually sodium or electrolytes). It is also important to drink plenty of cool water during exercise, about 7-10 oz. every 10-20 minutes during exercise. During exercise, sports drinks may be necessary to keep an electrolyte balance as well.

Dehydration-Mild: About 2% of water depletion	• Thirst • Decreased urine volume • Abnormally dark urine • Unexplained tiredness • Irritability • Lack of tears when crying • Headache • Dry mouth • Dizziness when standing due to orthostatic hypotension • May cause insomnia.
Moderate: About 5% -6%of water depletion	• Grogginess or sleepiness • Headache • Nausea • May feel tingling in limbs (parenthesis)
Severe: About 10% -15% of water depletion	• Muscles may become spastic • Skin may shrivel and wrinkle (decreased skin turgor) • Vision may dim • Urination will be greatly reduced and may become painful • Delirium may begin.
Over 15% of water depletion	• Usually, fatal.

COMPONENTS OF A CONDITIONING PROGRAM

WARM UP and COOL DOWN

Warming up and cooling down are very important parts of the exercise routine. There are physical and psychological benefits to both these components that can be as simple as a slow walk before and after your exercise program.

Benefits of warming up	Benefits of cooling down
<ul><li>Increases the temperature in the muscles, which increases the speed of contraction and relaxation.</li><li>Reduces premature lactic acid build up and fatigue during high level exercises.</li><li>Increases speed of nerve impulse conduction.</li><li>Increases elasticity of connective tissues</li><li>Increases muscle metabolism and oxygen consumption that enhances aerobic performance.</li><li>Alert for potential muscle injury that may arise during higher intensities.</li><li>Increases endorphins.</li><li>Allows the heart rate to get to a workable rate for beginning exercise.</li><li>Increases production of synovial fluid located between the joints to reduce friction.</li><li>Psychological warm up to mentally focus on training and competition.</li></ul>	<ul><li>Prevents venous blood pooling at the extremities, which reduces chance of dizziness or fainting.</li><li>Reduces the potential for Delayed Onset Muscle Soreness (DOMS).</li><li>Aids in removing waste products in muscles, such as lactic acid.</li><li>Reduces the level of adrenaline and other exercise hormones in the blood to lower the chance of post-exercise disturbances in cardiac rhythm.</li><li>Allows the heart to return back safely to resting rate.</li></ul>

Start out every routine with a warmup first. Here are some suggestions

- Walking or outside
- Running up and down some stairs
- Jumping jacks
- Running in place
- Dynamic stretching

Equipment

- Treadmill
- Stationary or Recumbent bike
- Stair climber or Elliptical
- Mini trampoline

Duration, Frequency, Intensity and Movement Patterns

Intensity: How *much* mental and physical *effort* it takes to sustain an activity.	This can be done using the target heart rate range THR (optimum exercise intensity levels through beats per minute, talk test or rate of perceived exertion.
Duration: How *long* the training lasts.	The higher the intensity, the shorter the duration. The American College of Sports Medicine guidelines recommends all healthy adults aged 18–65 yr should participate in moderate intensity aerobic physical activity for a minimum of 30 min on five days per week, or vigorous intensity aerobic activity for a minimum of 20 min on three days per week.
Frequency: How *often* the training occurs.	Training should be performed at least every other day or three days a week. Cardiac/aerobic conditioning can be done daily, although you may want to vary exercises. Regarding strength training, it is important to give each muscle group 48 hours to recover. Alternate upper and lower body with isolated abdomen/core exercises every other day. For those working out several days a week, find a schedule that works for you as long as you give each muscle group 48 hours of recovery time.
Movement Patterns and Examples Basic movements that help to increase overall body strengthening	<ul><li>Bend and Lift: Squats, Dead Lifts and Leg presses<ul><li>Picking up item off floor</li></ul></li><li>Single Leg: Step ups, Single leg stance, Lunges<ul><li>Walking up steps</li></ul></li><li>Push: Shoulder press, Bench press, Push up<ul><li>Pushing Shopping cart or Lawn mower</li></ul></li><li>Pull: Lat pull downs, Seated rows<ul><li>Vacuuming, Raking</li></ul></li><li>Rotational<ul><li>Shoveling snow</li></ul></li></ul>

Diaphragmatic Breathing

- Lie either on your back with your knees bent or sit up
- Inhale through your nose; as you do so, allow your stomach to rise. Limit movement in your chest. Attempt to push your bottom ribs out to the side as you breathe in.
- Exhale through your mouth; as you do so, allow your stomach to fall. Limit movement in your chest.
- Repeat for at least 10 cycles.

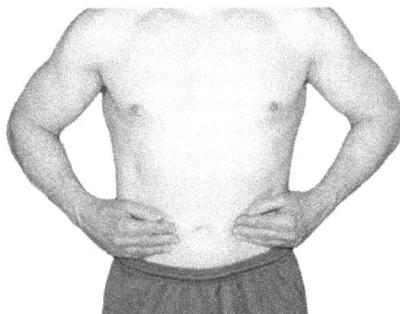

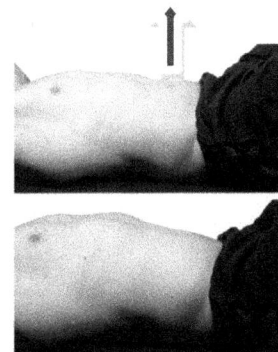

Pursed Lip Breathing

(PLB) is a breathing technique that consists of inhaling through the nose with the mouth closed and then exhaling through tightly pressed (pursed) lips. This technique is frequently in those with cardiac or respiratory issues.   *"Smell the Roses then Blow Out the Candle".*

Breathing with Exercise

Exhale on the exertion. For example, exhale when you are lying on your back and pushing a weight up or when bending your arm doing a bicep curl,. Inhale as you bring the weight slowly to your chest or when you straighten your arm with a bicep curl..

ANATOMY

ANATOMICAL POSITIONS and PLANES

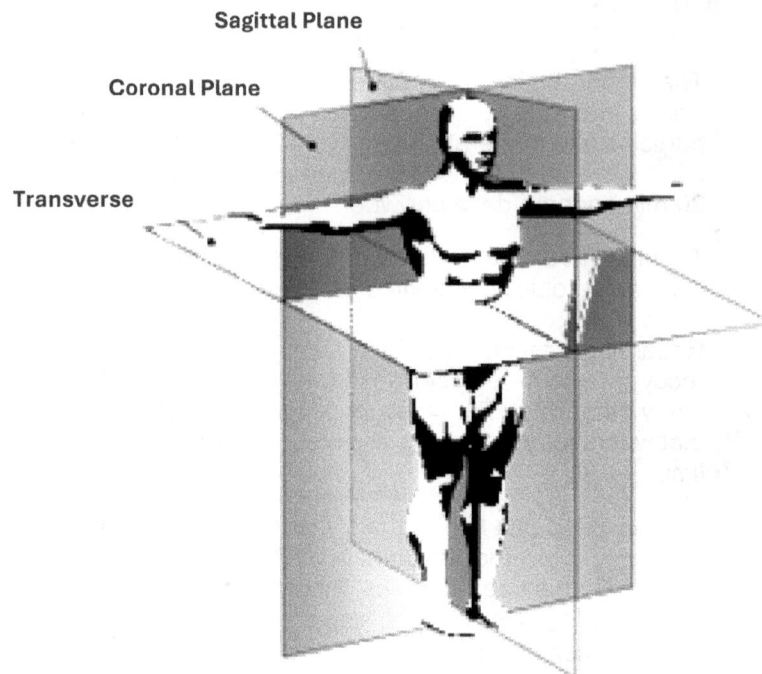

Anterior – Towards the front of the body.

Posterior – Towards the back of the body.

Distal – Away from the body or any point of reference, or from the point of attachment or origin.

Proximal – Closer to the body or any point of reference, or to the point of attachment or origin.

Medial – Situated towards the midline of the body.

Lateral – Position farther from the midline of the body.

Inferior – Away from the head or lower surface of a structure.

Superior – Towards the head or situated above.

Transverse /Axial / Horizontal plane is parallel to the ground, which separates the superior from the inferior or the head from the feet.

Coronal / Frontal/Frontal plane is perpendicular to the ground, which separates the anterior from the posterior or the front from the back

Sagittal / Lateral plane is a Y-Z plane, perpendicular to the ground, which separates left from right.

Upper Extremity (UE): Shoulders, Chest, Arms, Hands, etc

Lower Extremity (LE): Hips, Legs, Ankle Foot , etc

ANATOMICAL DIRECTIONS

Range of Motion (ROM): The distance and direction a joint can move between the flexed and extended position (*see flexion and extension below*). This can also be the act of attempting to increase the distance through therapeutic exercise and/or stretching for physiological gain.

Flexion - Bending movement that decreases the angle between two parts. Bending the knee or elbow are examples of flexion. Flexion of the hip or shoulder moves the limb forward (towards the front of the body).

Extension - The opposite of flexion; a straightening movement that increases the angle between body parts. The knees are extended when standing up. When straightening the arm, the elbow is extended. Extension of the hip or shoulder moves the limb backward (towards the back of the body).

Hyperextension – Extending the joint beyond extension.

Abduction - A lateral movement that pulls a structure or part away from the midline of the body. Raising the arms to the sides is an example of abduction.

Adduction - A medial movement that pulls a structure or part towards the midline of the body, or towards the midline of a limb. Dropping the arms to the sides, or bringing the knees together, are examples of adduction.

Internal rotation (or *medial rotation*). Inward rotary movement around the axis of the bone. Internal rotation of the shoulder or hip would point the toes or the flexed forearm inwards (towards the midline).

External rotation (or *lateral rotation*). External rotary movement around the axis of the bone. It would turn the toes or the flexed forearm outwards (away from the midline).

Elevation - Movement in a superior direction. Shrugging or bringing the shoulders up is an example of elevation.

Depression - Movement in an inferior direction, the opposite of elevation. Pushing the shoulders down is an example of depression.

Pronation - Internal rotation the hand or foot to face downward or posterior. Pronating the foot is a combination of eversion and abduction.

Supination - External rotation of the hand or foot to face upward or anterior. Raising the inside or medial margin of the foot.

Dorsiflexion – Movement at the ankle of the foot superiorly towards the shin. The up position of tapping the foot.

Plantarflexion – Movement at the ankle of the foot inferiorly away from the shin. Pointing the foot downward.

Eversion – Moving the sole of the foot away from the median plane or outward.

Inversion - Moving the sole of the foot towards the median plane or inward.

Ipsilateral – Same side of the body

Contralateral – Opposite side of the body

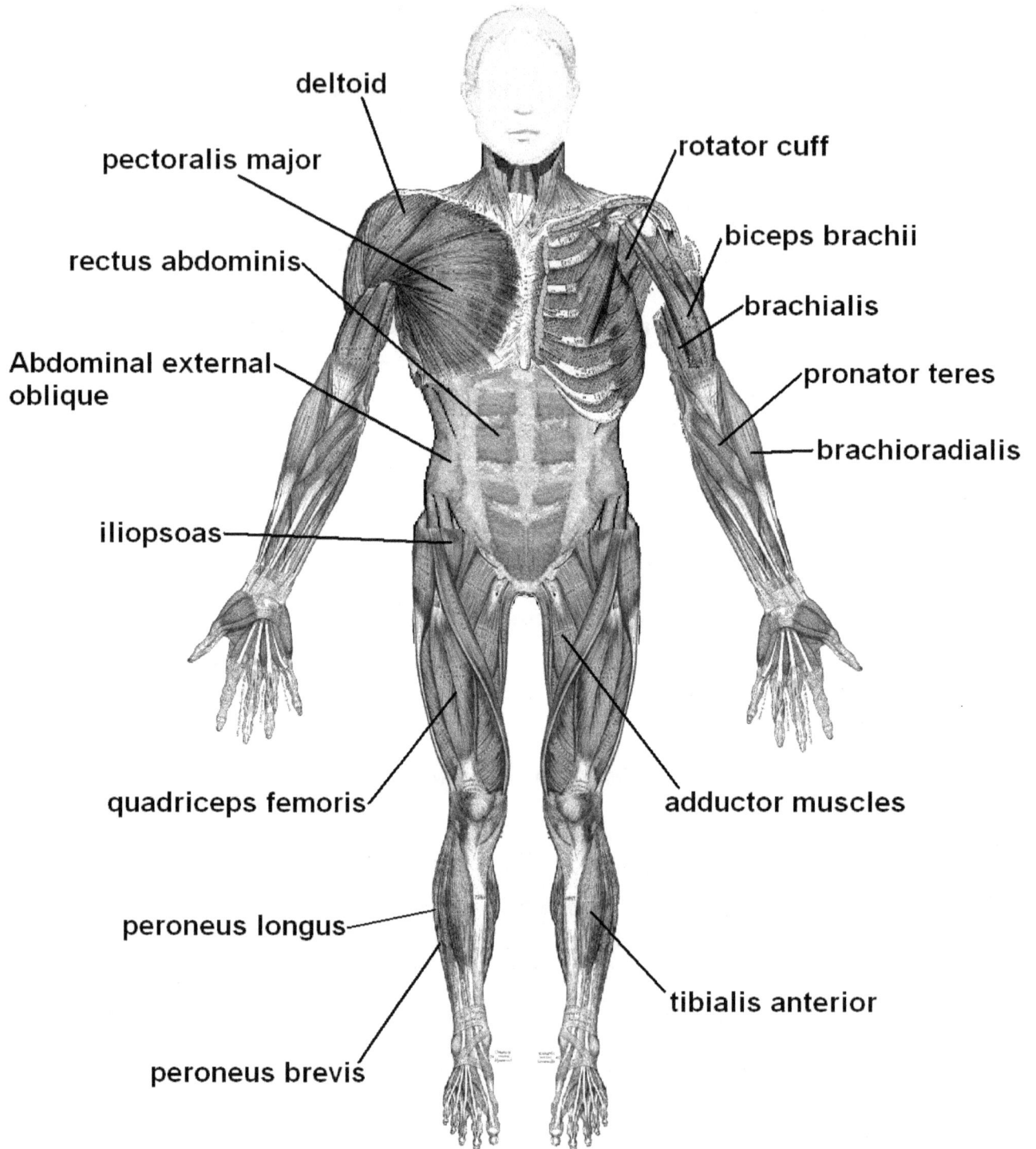

MUSCLES

Grey's Anatomy

ANTERIOR

deltoid

pectoralis major

rectus abdominis

Abdominal external oblique

iliopsoas

quadriceps femoris

peroneus longus

peroneus brevis

rotator cuff

biceps brachii

brachialis

pronator teres

brachioradialis

adductor muscles

tibialis anterior

Muscle Name (AKA)	Joint Action
Pectoralis major	Shoulder flexion, adduction, internal rotation
Deltoid (anterior)	Shoulder abduction, flexion, internal rotation
Rotator cuff (SITS) Supraspinatus Infraspinatus Teres minor Subscapularis	Shoulder: Supraspinatus: Abduction Infraspinatus: External rotation Teres minor: External rotation Subscapularis: Internal rotation
Biceps brachii	Elbow flexion; Forearm supination
Brachialis	Elbow flexion
Pronator teres	Elbow flexion; Forearm pronation
Brachioradialis	Elbow flexion
Tensor fasciae latae	Hip flexion, medial rotation & abduction
Gracilis*	Hip adduction & internal rotation;Knee flexion & internal rotation
Adductor muscles Adductor magnus, longus & brevis	Hip adduction
Tibialis anterior	Ankle dorsiflexion; foot inversion
Peroneus brevis	Ankle plantarflexion; Foot eversion
Peroneus longus	Ankle plantarflexion; Foot eversion
Rectus femoris (quadriceps femoris)	Hip extension (esp. when knee is extended); Knee flexion
Vastus medialis	Knee extension (esp. when hip is flexed)
Vastus lateralis	Knee extension (esp. when hip is flexed)
Sartorius	Hip flexion & external rotation; Knee flexion & internal rotation
Pectineus	Hip adduction
Iliopsoas, Psosas, Iliacus	Hip flexion & external rotation
Abdominal external oblique	Trunk lateral flexion
Rectus abdominis	Trunk flexion & lateral flexion
Abdominal internal oblique	Trunk lateral flexion

MUSCLES

Grey's Anatomy

POSTERIOR

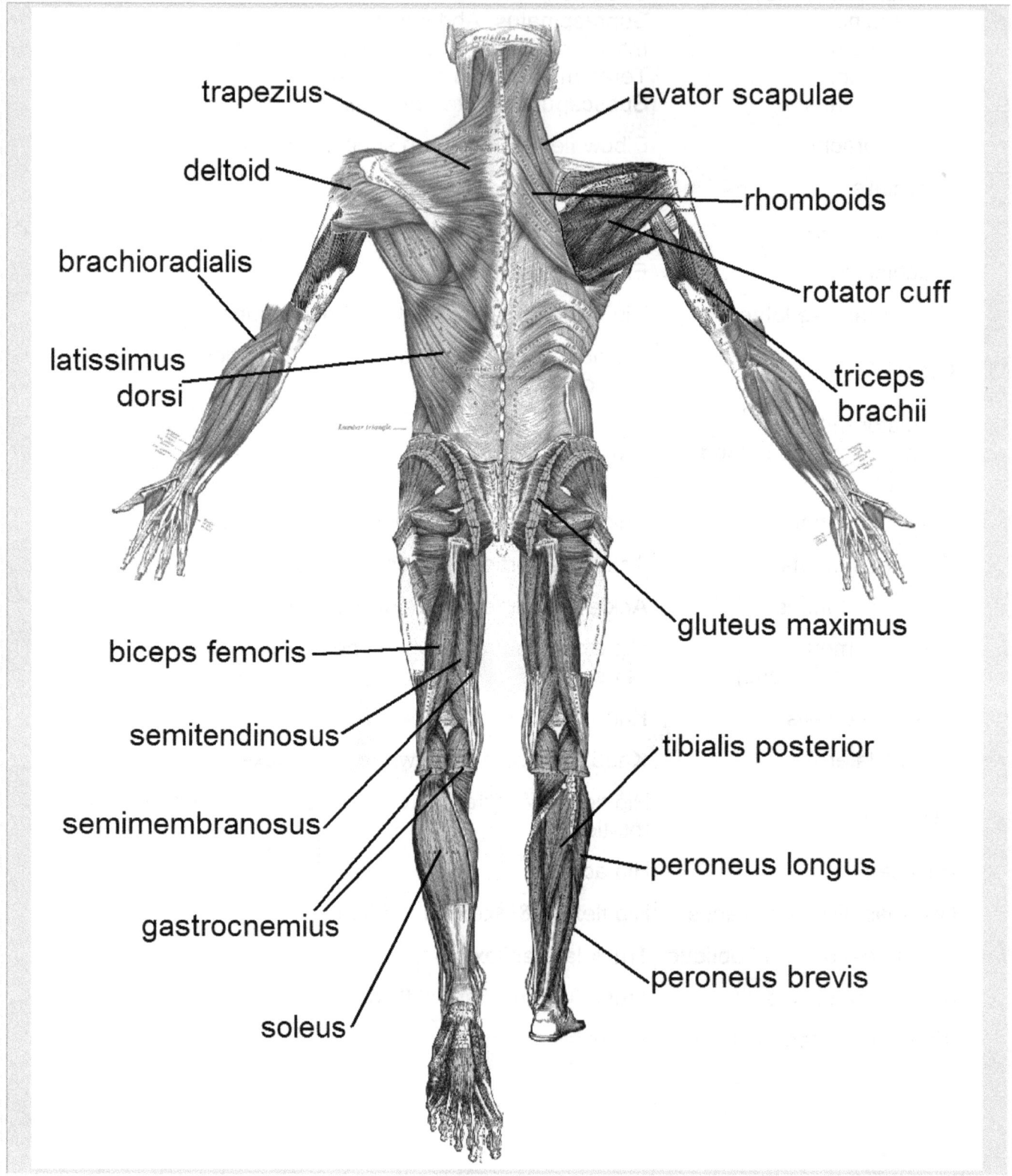

trapezius

levator scapulae

deltoid

rhomboids

brachioradialis

rotator cuff

latissimus dorsi

triceps brachii

gluteus maximus

biceps femoris

semitendinosus

tibialis posterior

semimembranosus

peroneus longus

gastrocnemius

peroneus brevis

soleus

Muscle Name (AKA)	Joint Action
Deltoid (posterior)	Shoulder abduction, extension, external rotation
Trapezius	Scapula or Shoulder girdle:, Upper traps: Scapula elevation. Middle traps: Scapula adduction. Lower traps: Scapula depression
Levator scapulae	Scapula elevation
Rhomboids	Scapula adduction & elevation
Triceps brachii	Elbow extension
Gluteus medius	Hip abduction
Gluteus maximus	Hip extension & external rotation
Tibialis, posterior	Inversion, stabilization, assists with plantarflexion
Soleus	Ankle plantarflexion
Gastrocnemius	Knee flexion; Ankle plantarflexion
Semimembranosus	Hip extension & internal rotation; Knee flexion & internal rotation
Semitendinosus	Hip extension & internal rotation; Knee flexion & internal rotation
Biceps femoris (long head)	Hip extension & internal rotation; Knee flexion & external rotation
Latissimus dorsi	Shoulder extension, adduction, internal rotation
Erector spinae, Longissimus, Spinalis, Iliocostalis	Trunk extension, hyperextension & lateral flexion Deep muscle that originate in the posterior iliac crest & sacrum running up the spine and inserts in the transverse process of ribs
Pes anserine, Gracilis, Sartorius, Semimembranosus, Semitendinosus	Internal rotation of tibia when knee is flexed

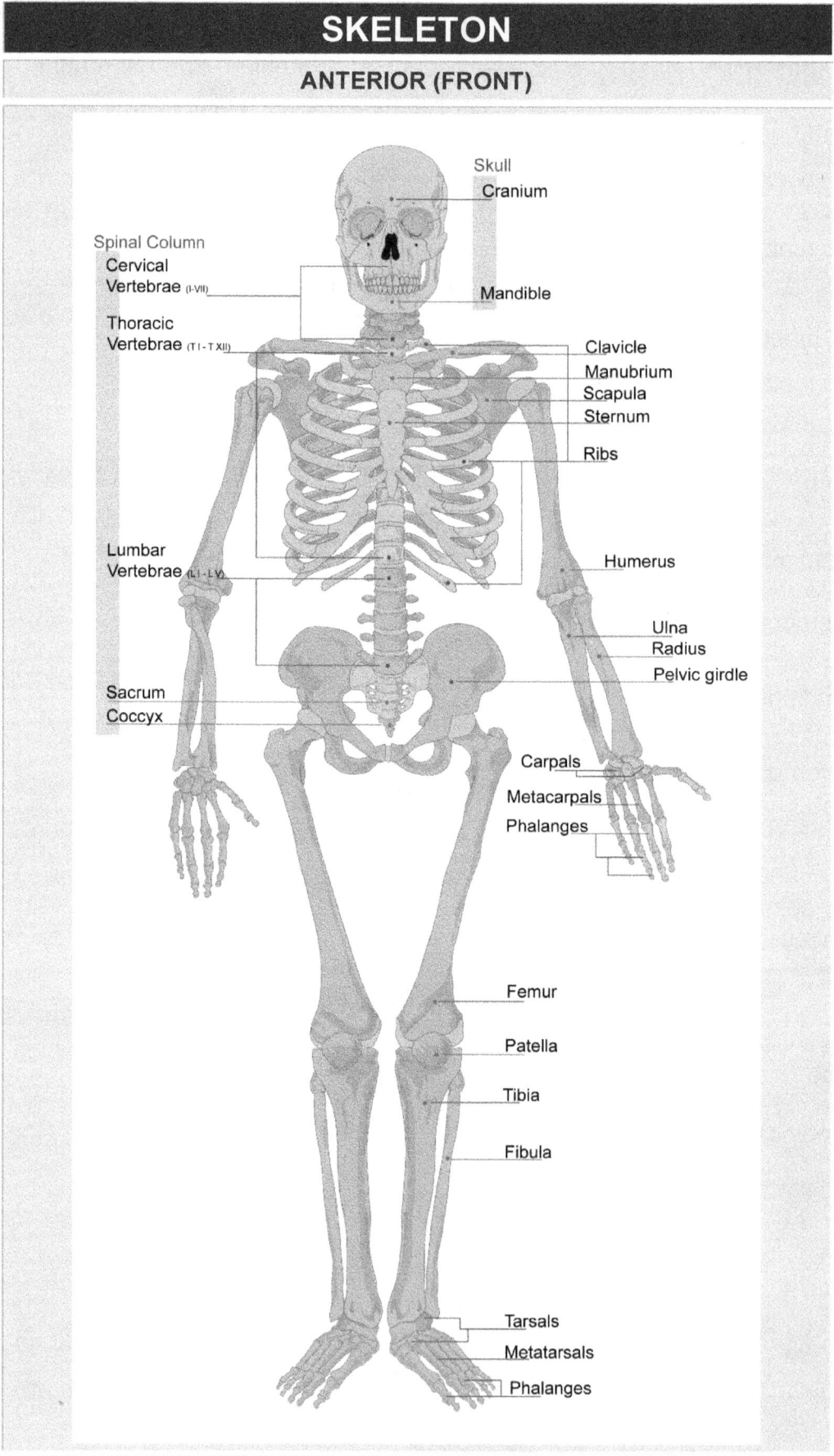

SKELETON

ANTERIOR (FRONT)

Skull
Cranium

Spinal Column
Cervical
Vertebrae (I-VII)

Mandible

Thoracic
Vertebrae (T I - T XII)

Clavicle
Manubrium
Scapula
Sternum

Ribs

Lumbar
Vertebrae (L I - L V)

Humerus

Ulna
Radius
Pelvic girdle

Sacrum
Coccyx

Carpals
Metacarpals
Phalanges

Femur

Patella

Tibia

Fibula

Tarsals
Metatarsals
Phalanges

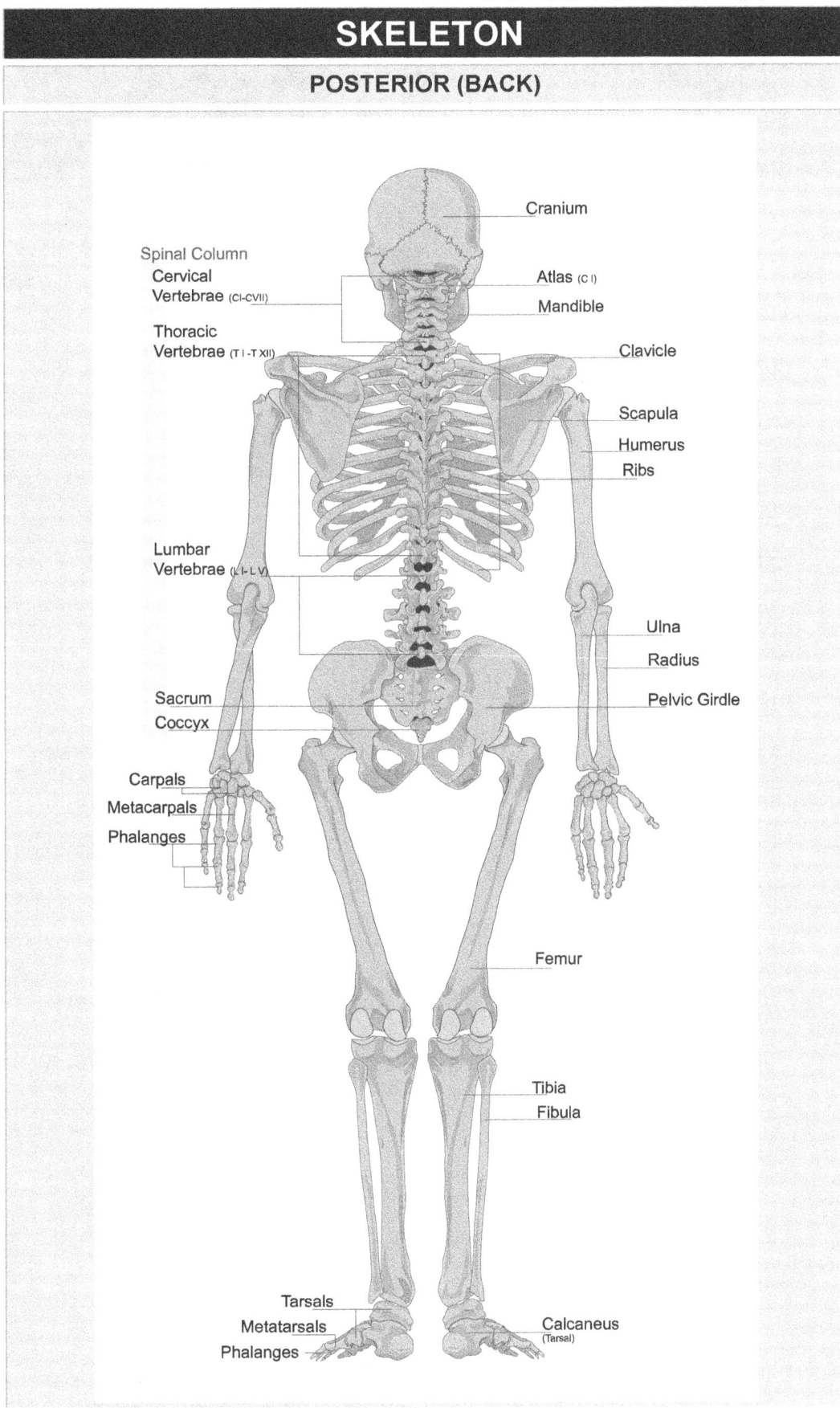

SKELETON

POSTERIOR (BACK)

Cranium

Spinal Column
Cervical
Vertebrae (CI-CVII)

Atlas (C I)

Mandible

Thoracic
Vertebrae (T I -T XII)

Clavicle

Scapula

Humerus

Ribs

Lumbar
Vertebrae (LI-LV)

Ulna

Radius

Sacrum

Coccyx

Pelvic Girdle

Carpals

Metacarpals

Phalanges

Femur

Tibia

Fibula

Tarsals

Metatarsals

Phalanges

Calcaneus
(Tarsal)

Average Joint Range of Motion

Anatomical Positions – Upper Extremity

Joint UPPER EXTREMITY	Movement	Normal Range of Motion (degrees)	Plane
Elbow	Flexion	150	Sagittal
	Extension	0 (neutral)	Sagittal
	Hyperextension	< 10	Sagittal
Shoulder	Flexion	180	Sagittal
	Extension	0 (neutral)	Sagittal
	Hyperextension	60	Sagittal
	Adduction (Add)	0 (neutral)	Frontal
	Abduction (Abd)	180	Frontal
	Horizontal Add/Flexion	130	Transverse
	Horizontal Abd	0 (to neutral)	Transverse
	Horizontal Extension	45	Transverse
	Internal rotation	70	Sagittal
	External rotation	90	Sagittal
Radioulnar	Pronation	90	Transverse
	Supination	90	Transverse

Average Joint Range of Motion

Anatomical Positions – Lower Extremity

Joint LOWER EXTREMITY	Movement	Normal Range of Motion (degrees)	Plane
Knee	Flexion	135	Sagittal
	Extension	0 (neutral)	Sagittal
	Hyperextension	10	Sagittal
Hip	Flexion	120	Sagittal
	Extension	0 (neutral)	Sagittal
	Hyperextension	< 20	Sagittal
	Adduction (Add)	0 (neutral)	Frontal
	Abduction (Abd)	50	Frontal
	Internal rotation	40	Transverse
	External rotation	50	Transverse
Ankle	Dorsiflexion	20	Sagittal
	Plantarflexion	50	Sagittal

EQUIPMENT used in this Book.

Don't buy a lot of equipment before knowing what your goals are.

Stability / Exercise Ball Bosu

These can replace an exercise bench if you do not have the space. It is also used for many of the core strengthening exercises

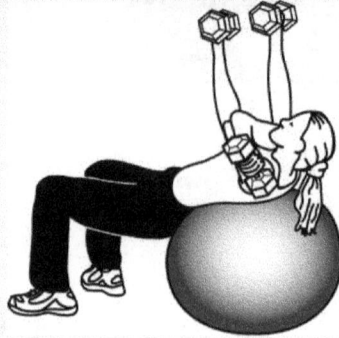

Should be inflated so that when you sit on it you are at a 90-degree angle.

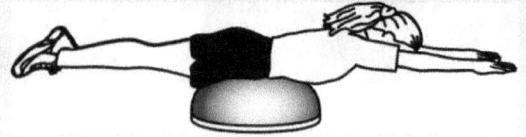

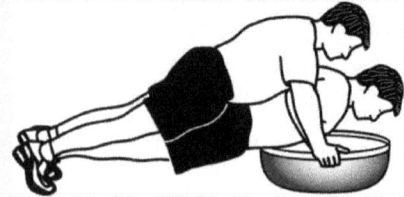

Dumbbells

Kettle Bell
(optional)

Dowel with/without weight

These will be needed for your strength exercises. See *Strengthening* section on for resistance.

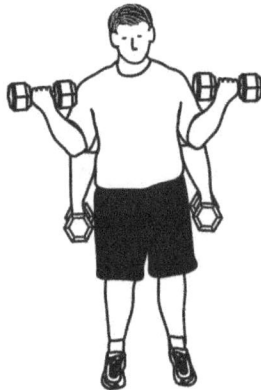

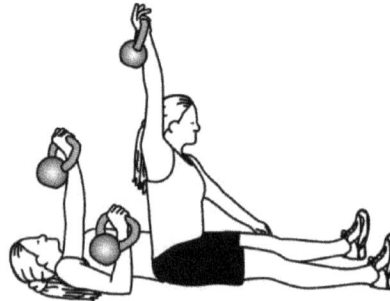

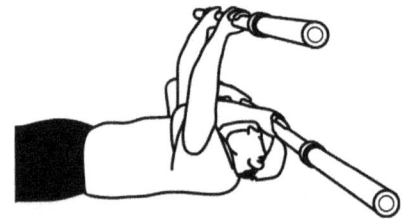

Resistance bands

In different weights/ resistance.

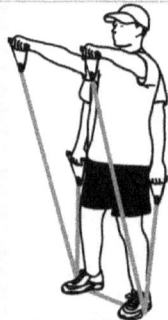

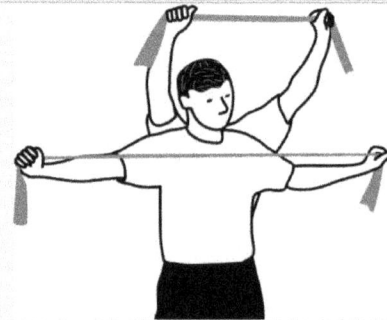

Agility Equipment

Cone hurdles, Speed hurdles, Agility ladder/rings/poles, Bosu, Stair step, Jump rope.

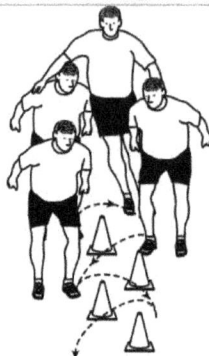

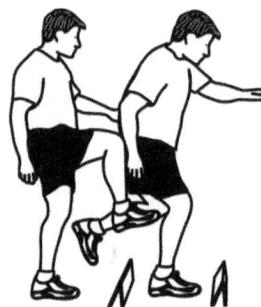

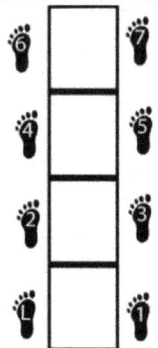

Balance Equipment

Can include **Foam rollers** *(also see Myofascial below)*

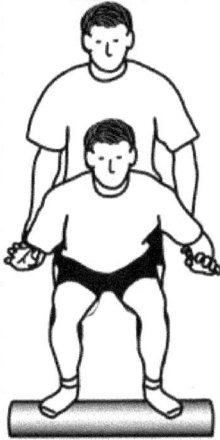

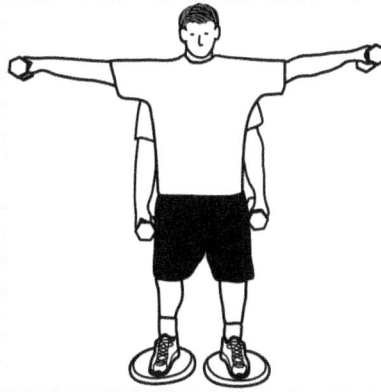

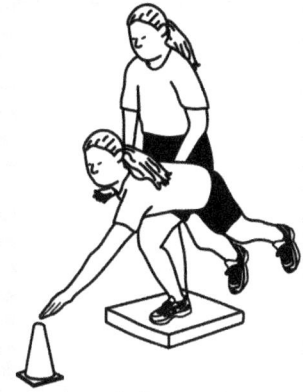

Balance discs
Balance pad
Cones
Stepper
Bosu

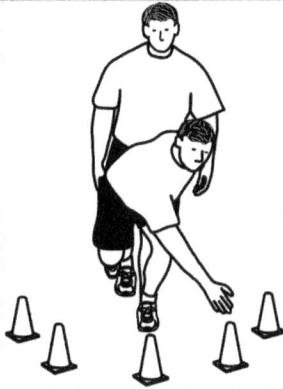

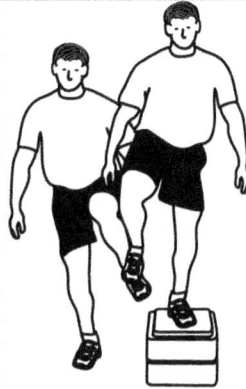

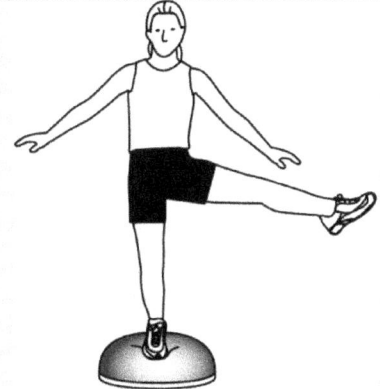

Exercise Bench (Optional)

The type really depends on what you will use it for. You can get a plain bench just for support (as above you can use a stability ball) or you can get all the bells and whistles. Some have pieces for leg extensions and curls, as well as arm pieces for butterflies. If you do not already have one, I suggest waiting until you start your exercise program and see what you feel you will need to advance.

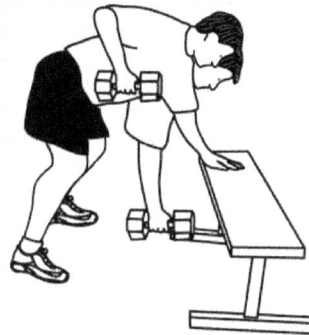

Examples For Myofascial

Massage Ball

Foam/Textured Rollers *(also see balance)*

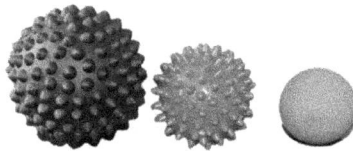

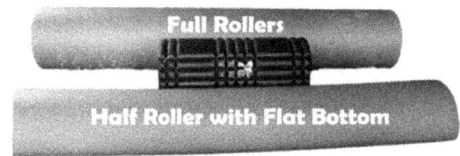

Full Rollers

Half Roller with Flat Bottom

Not Shown	• Exercise mat for floor exercises • Ankle Weights • Bed, couch or high table/mat • Chair with/without arms - High or Low	• 10-inch play ball • Pillow • Towel roll • Strap for stretches

SELF TESTS

Before starting the exercise program, it is a good idea to see where your baseline is. Taking the following tests will help guide you in the level you will need to start, and help progress by retaking the test periodically. *It is suggested to get a partner to help with both timing and safety, especially with balance tests.* The first 6 tests are modified versions starting at age 60 but are great for adults of any age. Tests 7-10 will help determine how quickly you can advance your balance program.

As with the exercises in this book, these tests should also be performed by those that are otherwise healthy with no chronic or acute ailments OR with supervision of a qualified health coach/personal trainer/physical therapist.

Tests 1-6 should be conducted in the following order if you are doing them at the same time.

A general warm up should be done prior to tests (*see Warm up/Cool down*).
- Stop immediately if any adverse reactions, such as nausea, dizziness, blurred vision, pain of any kind, chest pain, confusion or loss of muscle control.
- Stay hydrated, and do not proceed with testing on days with high temperature/humidity or any other conditions where you would not normally exercise.
- Practice each test several times before attempting to get an accurate score.
- It is advised that you have a second person to time the tests and make sure you are following proper form. Make sure your partner also understands the precautions and goals of these tests.

1. 30 second chair stand - Lower body strength
   o Needed for stair climbing, walking getting up out of tub/chair/car and reduce the risk of falls
2. 30 second arm curl test – Upper body strength
   o Needed to lift and carry everyday items, such as groceries and toolbox
3. 2-minute step test – Aerobic endurance
   o Needed for activities that require endurance, such as walking distance, grocery shopping and climbing stairs
4. Chair sit and reach – Lower body flexibility
   o Needed for normal gait patterns, correct posture, getting in/out of car/tub
5. Back stretch test – Shoulder flexibility
   o Needed to do various activities, such as combing hair and putting on overhead garments
6. 8 foot get up and go – Agility and dynamic balance
   o Needed for pretty much anything you do that requires getting up and walking, such as go to kitchen, bathroom or answering phone.
7. Narrow stance – Balance progression
8. Staggered stance – Balance progression
9. Tandem stance – Balance progression
10. One leg standing – Balance progression

TEST AND PURPOSE	PICTURE	EQUIPMENT NEEDED	EXPLANATION	RESULTS
30 Second Chair Stand Assess lower body strength *May not want to perform if any chronic pain or back issues. *If you are tall and have had a recent hip replacement skip this or use taller chair.		Straight back or folding chair (~17 inch height) against wall. Stopwatch, wrist watch or clock within view with second hand	*Sit with feet flat on the floor and arms crossed over the chest. *Get up to a full stand and then sit back down. ** Start the time – Immediately repeat as many *full stands* as you can in 30 seconds. *If you cannot stand with hands over chest, try pushing off on your thighs or get a chair with arms and push off arms. If using assist, make sure you note this for progression.*	**Normal Range repetitions** <table><tr><td>Age</td><td>Men</td><td>Women</td></tr><tr><td>60-64</td><td>14-19</td><td>12-17</td></tr><tr><td>65-69</td><td>12-18</td><td>11-16</td></tr><tr><td>70-74</td><td>12-17</td><td>10-15</td></tr><tr><td>75-79</td><td>11-17</td><td>10-15</td></tr><tr><td>80-84</td><td>10-15</td><td>9-14</td></tr><tr><td>85-89</td><td>8-14</td><td>8-13</td></tr><tr><td>90-94</td><td>7-12</td><td>4-11</td></tr></table>
TEST AND PURPOSE	PICTURE	EQUIPMENT NEEDED	EXPLANATION	RESULTS
30 Second Arm Curl Test Upper body strength		Straight back or folding chair without arms. Can be done in standing. Stopwatch or clock within view with second hand Women: 5 lb dumbbell Men: 8 lb dumbbell Can use a wrist weight if arthritis and cannot hold a dumbbell	*Sit with feet flat on the floor towards the edge seat towards dominant side. **Start with the arm extended by your side holding dumbbell in the dominant hand. *Bend elbow with palm facing you keeping the upper arm next to the body (elbow pressed into your side). *Return to starting position. *Keep the wrist straight – do not flex or extend the wrist. **Start the time – Immediately repeat as many arm curls as you can in 30 seconds *with proper form.* *If you cannot hold the suggested weight with proper form, use a lighter weight. Make sure you note this for progression.*	**Normal Range repetitions** <table><tr><td>Age</td><td>Men</td><td>Women</td></tr><tr><td>60-64</td><td>16-22</td><td>13-19</td></tr><tr><td>65-69</td><td>15-21</td><td>12-18</td></tr><tr><td>70-74</td><td>14-21</td><td>12-17</td></tr><tr><td>75-79</td><td>13-19</td><td>11-17</td></tr><tr><td>80-84</td><td>13-19</td><td>10-16</td></tr><tr><td>85-89</td><td>11-17</td><td>10-15</td></tr><tr><td>90-94</td><td>10-14</td><td>8-13</td></tr></table>

TEST AND PURPOSE	PICTURE	EQUIPMENT NEEDED	EXPLANATION	RESULTS
2 Minute Step Test Aerobic endurance		Wall for support and to mark step height. Sturdy chair to hold on opposite side if unsteady. Stopwatch or clock within view with second hand	*For accuracy, may need a second person to judge step height and count. *Step with side next to wall. Bring knee up mid-thigh between the knee and the hip. Mark the wall with tape at this height. This will be your minimum step height. *Practice marching in place to this step height. **Start the time – Immediately start marching (not jogging) for 2 minutes. Count the number of *full steps* (both legs) that come up to step height. Every time the right knee reaches proper step height; this is counted as one step. **If shortness of breath, extreme fatigue or unable to continue to step height, stop test and this is your baseline.* ** If unable to get to step height, but able to complete 2 minutes. Make sure you note this for progression.* **If unsteady, hold onto chair on opposite side for support.*	**Normal Range steps** | Age	Men	Women
---	---	---
60-64	87-115	75-107
65-69	86-116	73-107
70-74	80-110	68-101
75-79	73-109	68-100
80-84	71-103	60-90
85-89	59-91	55-85
90-94	52-86	44-72	

TEST AND PURPOSE	PICTURE	EQUIPMENT NEEDED	EXPLANATION	RESULTS
Chair Sit And Reach Lower body flexibility, *primarily hamstrings* *Do not do if recent hip replacement or severe osteoporosis. *Stretch to discomfort, not pain.		Chair (~17 inch height). Make sure chair is secure and does not tip forward. 18 inch ruler or yardstick	*Sit on the edge chair – you should feel the middle of the thigh at the edge of the chair. *Bend one leg with foot flat on floor. *Straighten the target leg in front with heel on the floor and foot flexed up. *Reach forward with one hand over the other and middle fingers even. *Exhale as you bend forward at the hips and reach forward towards or past the toes. Keep the extended knee straight and adjust if it bends. *Practice a few times on both legs to see which one you would prefer for testing. Do two tests and measure as below. **Measure tips of middle fingers to the tip of the shoe (closest to ½ inch). ***The midpoint at the toe of the shoe is considered zero (0), and is scored as such if you reach this point. ***If the reach is short, score this as a minus (-) ***If the reach is past this point, score this as a plus (+)	See table below

Normal Range inches (Chair Sit And Reach)

Age	Men	Women
60-64	-2.5 +4.0	-0.5 + 5.0
65-69	-3.0 +3.0	-0.5 + 4.5
70-74	-3.0 +3.0	-1.0 + 4.0
75-79	-4.0 +2.0	-1.5 + 3.5
80-84	-5.5 +1.5	2.0 + 3.0
85-89	-5.5 +0.5	-2.5 + 2.5
90-94	-6.5 -0.5	-4.5 + 1.0

TEST AND PURPOSE	PICTURE	EQUIPMENT NEEDED	EXPLANATION	RESULTS
Back Stretch Test Shoulder flexibility *Do not do if any upper back, shoulder or neck injuries		18-inch ruler or yardstick	*Will need second person to measure. *Stand and place the target arm over the same shoulder, palm down with fingers extended. Reach down the middle of the back. *Place the opposite arm around the back, palm up reaching up the middle of the back towards other hand. Try to touch middle fingers together or overlap if possible. *Do not overlap fingers and pull.* *Practice a few times on both arms to see which one you would prefer for testing. Do two tests and measure as below. **Measure the distance between tips of middle fingers or overlap. ***If the middle fingers do not touch, score this as a minus (-) ***If the middle fingers just touch, score this as a zero (0) ***If the middle fingers overlap, score this as a plus (+)	See table below

Normal Range inches (Back Stretch Test)

Age	Men	Women
60-64	-6.5 +0.0	-3.0 + 1.5
65-69	-7.5 -1.0	-3.5 + 1.5
70-74	-8.0 -1.0	-4.0 + 1.0
75-79	-9.0 -2.0	-5.0 + 0.5
80-84	-9.5 -2.0	-5.5 + 0.0
85-89	-9.5 -3.0	-7.0 -1.0
90-94	-10.5 -4.0	-8.0 -1.0

TEST AND PURPOSE	PICTURE	EQUIPMENT NEEDED	EXPLANATION	RESULTS		
8 Foot Get Up And Go Agility and dynamic balance *If unsteady, have someone by your side in case you lose your balance.		Chair against wall (~17-inch height) Cone or another marker to walk around Stopwatch or clock within view with second hand *Put chair against wall and cone 8 feet in front. Measure from front of chair to back of cone (side facing chair).	*This is done better with a partner watching the clock or a stopwatch. *Sit on chair, back straight, feet flat on floor, one foot slightly in front, torso leaning slightly forward and hands resting on thighs. **Start the time – Immediately get up and walk around the cone (either side) and return to chair. Stopwatch immediately when seated. **Try 2-3x and record the fastest time within 10th /second. *Can use a cane or walker or start from standing position. Make sure you note this for progression.	**Normal Range seconds**		

				Age	Men	Women
				60-64	5.6-3.8	6.0-4.4
				65-69	5.9-4.3	6.4-4.8
				70-74	6.2-4.4	7.1-4.9
				75-79	7.2-4.6	7.4-5.2
				80-84	7.6-5.2	8.7-5.7
				85-89	8.9-5.5	9.6-6.2
				90-94	10.0-6.2	11.5-7.3

(8 feet →)

TEST AND PURPOSE	PICTURE	EQUIPMENT NEEDED	EXPLANATION	RESULTS
Narrow Stance Balance progression		Wall, counter or chair within arm's reach for support if needed Stopwatch or clock within view with second hand	Keep your feet together and stand for up to one minute. *Time stops if loss of balance with need to hold on to support.	One minute: Normal *Progress to Staggered Stance Test* *Less than 30 seconds: Continue balance program with wider stance and progress to narrow stance using support. *(See Balance)*
Staggered Stance Balance progression		Wall, counter or chair within arm's reach for support if needed Stopwatch or clock within view with second hand	Stand with one foot in front of the other and slightly off to the side. Stand for up to one minute. Repeat on other side for comparison *Time stops if loss of balance with need to hold on to support.	One minute: Normal *Progress to Tandem Stance Test* *Less than 30 seconds: Continue balance program using support. *(See Balance)*
Tandem Stance Balance progression		Wall, counter or chair within arm's reach for support if needed Stopwatch or clock within view with second hand	Stand with one foot directly in back of the other – toe should be touching the opposite heel. Hold for up to one minute. Repeat on other side for comparison *Time stops if loss of balance with need to hold on to support.	One minute: Normal *Progress to One Leg Standing Balance* *Less than 30 seconds: Continue balance program using support. *(See Balance)*
Single Leg Stance Balance progression		Wall, counter or chair within arm's reach for support if needed Stopwatch or clock within view with second hand	Stand on one leg for up to one minute. Repeat on other side for comparison *Time stops if loss of balance with need to hold on to support or if opposite foot taps the floor	One minute: Normal *Less than 30 seconds: Continue balance program using support. *(See Balance)*

EXERCISE **Myofascial Release**	EXERCISE NUMBER	PAGE	REPS	SETS	X DAY	HOLD
ANTERIOR CHEST - BALL	1					
ANTERIOR CHEST - FOAM ROLL	2					
LATISSIMUS DORSI – BALL	3					
LATISSIMUS DORSI - FOAM ROLL	4					
TRICEP – FOAM ROLL	5					
OCCIPITAL RELEASE - FOAM ROLL	6					
THORACIC MOBILIZATION – SUPINE - FOAM ROLL	7					
THORACIC MOBILIZATION – STANDING - FOAM ROLL	8					
LUMBAR – STANDING – BALL - can do with foam roll	9					
LUMBAR – SUPINE – FOAM ROLLER	10					
HIP FLEXORS - BALL	11					
HIP FLEXORS – FOAM ROLL	12					
QUADRICEPS – BILATERAL - FOAM ROLL	13					
QUADRICEP – SINGLE - FOAM ROLL	14					
GLUTE /PIRIFORMIS - FOAM ROLL	15					
HIP ADDUCTORS – FOAM ROLL	16					
HAMSTRING – BILATERAL - FOAM ROLL	17					
HAMSTRING – SINGLE – FOAM ROLL	18					
CALVES – BILATERAL - FOAM ROLL	19					
CALVES – SINGLE - FOAM ROLL	20					
ILIOTIBIAL BAND (IT Band) - FOAM ROLL	21					
ILIOTIBIAL BAND (IT Band) - BALL	22					
PLANTAR FASCIA ROLLING – BALL	23					
PLANTAR FASCIA ROLLING - COLD SODA CAN	24					

EXERCISE Flexibility (Stretching)	EXERCISE NUMBER	PAGE	REPS	SETS	X DAY	HOLD
INVERSION	1					
EVERSION	2					
ANTERIOR TIBIALIS	3					
PLANTARFLEXION	4					
DORSIFLEXION - STRAP	5					
DORSIFLEXION - FLOOR ASSISTED	6					
STANDING CALF STRETCH - GASTROC	7					
STANDING CALF STRETCH - GASTROC – HAND ON KNEE	8					
GASTROCNEMIUS STAIR STRETCH	9					
STANDING CALF STRETCH - SOLEUS	10					
HAMSTRING STRETCH – TOWEL, BAND, STRAP or BELT	11					
HAMSTRING STRETCH – TOWEL, BAND, STRAP or BELT	12					
HAMSTRING STRETCH - TABLE, BED OR COUCH	13					
HAMSTRING / KNEE EXTENSION STRETCH - SEATED	14					
HAMSTRING STRETCH - STANDING	15					
TOE TOUCH – STANDING - NARROW or WIDE BOS	16					
HEEL SLIDES - SELF ASSISTED	17					
HEEL SLIDES - LONG SIT ASSISTED - TOWEL, BAND, STRAP or BELT	18					
HEEL SLIDES - SUPINE	19					
KNEE BENDS - EXERCISE BALL	20					
KNEE FLEXION – SELF ASSISTED - PRONE	21					
KNEE FLEXION – BELT ASSISTED - PRONE	22					
HEEL SLIDES - SELF ASSISTED	23					
HEEL SLIDES - SEATED	24					
KNEE FLEXION – SCOOT FORWARD - SEATED	25					

EXERCISE Flexibility (Stretching)	EXERCISE NUMBER	PAGE	REPS	SETS	X DAY	HOLD
KNEE FLEXION – STAIR OR STEP	26					
PIRIFORMIS STRETCH	27					
PIRIFORMIS STRETCH - EXERCISE BALL	28					
PIRIFORMIS STRETCH - LONG SIT	29					
PIRIFORMIS STRETCH – STANDING	30					
HIP FLEXOR STRETCH - SIDE OF BALL or CHAIR	31					
HIP FLEXOR STRETCH - STANDING	32					
HIP FLEXOR STRETCH - HALF KNEEL	33					
RUNNER'S STRETCH - MODIFIED	34					
HIP FLEXOR STRETCH – SUPINE	35					
HIP FLEXOR STRETCH – SUPINE - 2	36					
QUAD STRETCH - SIDELYING	37					
QUAD STRETCH - STANDING	38					
KNEE FALL OUT STRETCH or FROG STRETCH	39					
BUTTERFLY STRETCH	40					
HIP ADDUCTOR STRECH – KNEELING	41					
HIP ADDUCTOR STRECH - STANDING	42					
HIP EXTERNAL ROTATION STRETCH - SUPINE	43					
HIP INTERNAL ROTATION STRETCH - SEATED	44					
IT BAND STRETCH - STANDING	45					
IT BAND STRETCH -- SIDELYING	46					
NECK ROTATION and SIDE BENDS	47					
NECK FLEXION AND EXTENSION	48					
TRUNK FLEXION - SEATED	49					
LOW BACK STRETCH - SEATED	50					
LOW BACK STRETCH – STANDING - STRAIGHT & LATERAL	51					
LOW BACK STRETCH – RAIL OR DOORKNOB	52					

EXERCISE Flexibility (Stretching)	EXERCISE NUMBER	PAGE	REPS	SETS	X DAY	HOLD
PRAYER STRETCH and LATERAL	53					
PRAYER STRETCH - EXERCISE BALL	54					
CAT AND CAMEL	55					
KNEE TO CHEST STRETCH - SINGLE and BILATERAL	56					
PRONE ON ELBOWS	57					
PRESS UPS	58					
TRUNK ROTATION STRETCH – SINGLE LEG	59					
LOWER TRUNK ROTATIONS – BILATERAL	60					
TRUNK ROTATION - SEATED	61					
TRUNK ROTATION - STANDING or SEATED – DOWEL	62					
LATERAL TRUNK STRETCH - SINGLE, SEATED or STANDING	63					
LATERAL TRUNK STRETCH - BILATERAL SEATED or STANDING	64					
FLEXION - SUPINE - DOWEL	65					
WALL WALK	66					
FLEXION - TABLE SLIDE	67					
FLEXION - TABLE SLIDE - BALL	68					
EXTERNAL ROTATION - SUPINE – DOWEL *INTERNAL ROTATION ON OPPOSITE ARM*	69					
EXTERNAL ROTATION - 90-90 - DOWEL	70					
EXTERNAL ROTATION – SEATED – DOWEL *INTERNAL ROTATION ON OPPOSITE ARM*	71					
EXTERNAL ROTATION – STANDING – DOWEL *INTERNAL ROTATION ON OPPOSITE ARM*	72					
ABDUCTION - TABLE SLIDE - BALL	75					
ABDUCTION WITH DOWEL	76					
LYING DOWN EXTENSION - TABLE or BED	77					
WAND EXTENSION - STANDING	78					
CHEST STRETCH – SEATED, STANDING, or SUPINE	79					

Worksheets

EXERCISE Flexibility (Stretching)	EXERCISE NUMBER	PAGE	REPS	SETS	X DAY	HOLD
TRICEP STRETCH - STRAP or TOWEL	82					
POSTERIOR SHOULDER/DELTOID RELEASE	83					
POSTERIOR CAPSULE STRETCH	84					

Worksheets

EXERCISE Core / Stability	EXERCISE NUMBER	PAGE	REPS	SETS	X DAY	HOLD
ABDOMINAL BRACING TRAINING	1					
ABDOMINAL BRACING - SUPINE	2					
PELVIC TILT - SUPINE	3					
PELVIC TILT - KNEELING	4					
BRIDGING	5					
BRIDGE - BOSU	6					
BRIDGING WITH PILLOW SQUEEZE	7					
BRIDGING WITH PILLOW SQUEEZE - BOSU	8					
BRACE SUPINE MARCHING / BRIDGE LEG UP	9					
BRIDGE LEG UP - BOSU -	10					
SINGLE LEG BRIDGE	11					
BRIDGE SINGLE LEG - BOSU	12					
BRIDGING CROSSED LEG	13					
BRIDGING CROSSED LEG – BOSU	14					
BRIDGING CROSSED LEG - ARMS UP	15					
BRIDGING CROSSED LEG - ARMS UP - BOSU	16					
BRIDGE - ELASTIC BAND	17					
BRIDGING - ABDUCTION - ELASTIC BAND	18					
FLOOR BRIDGE - EXERCISE BALL	19					
FLOOR BRIDGE ALTERNATE LEG LIFT - EXERCISE BALL	20					
BRIDGE UPPER BACK - EXERCISE BALL	21					
BRIDGE UPPER BACK - SINGLE LEG - EXERCISE BALL	22					
QUADRUPED ALTERNATE ARM	23					
QUADRUPED ALTERNATE LEG	24					
QUADRUPED ALTERNATE ARM AND LEG	25					
BIRD DOG ELBOW TOUCHES	26					

EXERCISE Core / Stability	EXERCISE NUMBER	PAGE	REPS	SETS	X DAY	HOLD
PRONE BALL	27					
PRONE BALL - ALTERNATE ARM	28					
PRONE BALL - ALTERNATE LEG	29					
PRONE BALL - ALTERNATE ARM AND LEG	30					
MODIFIED PLANK	31					
MODIFIED PLANK - ALTERNATE LEG	32					
FULL PLANK	33					
PLANK - ALTERNATE ARMS	34					
PLANK - ALTERNATE LEGS	35					
PLANK - EXERCISE BALL	36					
PRONE ON ELBOWS	37					
PRESS UPS	38					
SKYDIVER	39					
PRONE SUPERMAN - BOSU	40					
TRUNK EXTENSION - BOSU	41					
TRUNK EXTENSION - HANDS CROSSED IN FRONT - BOSU	43					
SUPERMAN - ARMS BACK- EXERCISE BALL	44					
SUPERMAN – BOTH ARMS IN FRONT - EXERCISE BALL	45					
SUPERMAN – ONE ARM FORWARD / ONE ARM BACK - EXERCISE BALL	46					
LATERAL PLANK MODIFIED	47					
LATERAL PLANK MODIFIED- BOSU	48					
LATERAL PLANK - 1 KNEE 1 FOOT	49					
LATERAL PLANK - 1 KNEE 1 FOOT – BOSU	50					
LATERAL PLANK	51					
LATERAL PLANK - BOSU	52					

EXERCISE Core / Stability	EXERCISE NUMBER	PAGE	REPS	SETS	X DAY	HOLD
LEAN BACK	53					
LEAN BACK - BOSU	54					
LEAN BACK WITH ARMS OUT	55					
LEAN BACK WITH ARMS OUT - BOSU	56					
LEAN BACK WITH TWIST	57					
LEAN BACK WITH TWIST – BOSU	58					
CRUNCHY FROG	59					
SEATED BIKE - FORWARD AND BACKWARDS	60					
CRUNCH – ARMS OUT	61					
CRUNCH – ARMS OUT - BOSU	62					
CRUNCH – ARMS IN BACK OF HEAD	63					
CRUNCH – ARMS IN BACK OF HEAD - BOSU	64					
OBLIQUE CRUNCH	65					
OBLIQUE CRUNCH - BOSU	66					
90 DEGREE CRUNCH	67					
BALL CRUNCH – Can put legs on seat of chair	68					
CURL UPS – ARMS ON LEGS - EXERCISE BALL	69					
CURL UPS- ARMS CROSSED IN FRONT - EXERCISE BALL	70					
CURL UPS – ARMS BEHIND HEAD - EXERCISE BALL	71					
SUPINE CRUNCH TOUCH - EXERCISE BALL	72					
LOWER ABDOMINAL CRUNCH – WITH or WITHOUT BALL	73					
HIGH MARCH CRUNCH	74					
STANDING SIDE CRUNCH	75					
STANDING BIKE CRUNCH	76					

EXERCISE Lower Extremity - Lying & Seated Strengthening and Range of Motion	EXERCISE NUMBER	PAGE	REPS	SETS	X DAY	HOLD
INVERSION – SEATED - ELASTIC BAND	1					
INVERSION – SEATED - ELASTIC BAND - 2	2					
EVERSION – SEATED - ELASTIC BAND	3					
EVERSION – SEATED - ELASTIC BAND - 2	4					
ANKLE PUMPS - SEATED	5					
ANKLE PUMPS – SUPINE or FEET UP ON STOOL	6					
DORSIFLEXION – SEATED - ELASTIC BAND	7					
DORSIFLEXION – SEATED - ELASTIC BAND - 2	8					
PLANTARFLEXION - STRAP	9					
PLANTARFLEXION - SEATED – ELASTIC BAND	10					
HEEL SLIDES - SUPINE	11					
HEEL SLIDES - RESISTED EXTENSION – ELASTIC BAND	12					
QUAD SET –ISOMETRIC	13					
QUAD SET WITH TOWEL UNDER HEEL - ISOMETRIC	14					
SHORT ARC QUAD (SAQ) – SELF ASSISTED	15					
SHORT ARC QUAD - (SAQ)	16					
KNEE EXTENSION - SELF ASSISTED	17					
PARTIAL ARC QUAD - LOW SEAT	18					
LONG ARC QUAD (LAQ) – LOW SEAT (90 deg)	19					
LONG ARC QUAD (LAQ) – LOW SEAT - ANKLE WEIGHTS	20					
LONG ARC QUAD (LAQ) - HIGH SEAT	21					
LONG ARC QUAD (LAQ) - HIGH SEAT - ANKLE WEIGHTS	22					
LONG ARC QUAD - ELASTIC BAND – HAND HELD	23					
LONG ARC QUAD - ELASTIC BAND	24					

Worksheets

EXERCISE Lower Extremity - Lying & Seated Strengthening and Range of Motion	EXERCISE NUMBER	PAGE	REPS	SETS	X DAY	HOLD
HAMSTRING CURLS - PRONE - ASSISTED	25					
HAMSTRING CURLS - PRONE	26					
HAMSTRING CURLS - - PRONE - WEIGHTS	27					
HAMSTRING CURLS – PRONE - ELASTIC BAND	28					
HAMSTRING CURLS – ELASTIC BAND	29					
HAMSTRING CURLS – ELASTIC BAND - 2	30					
HAMSTRING CURLS ON BALL	31					
HAMSTRING CURLS - SINGLE LEG - EXERCISE BALL	32					
HIP FLEXION ISOMETRIC	33					
HIP FLEXION ISOMETRIC BILATERAL	34					
HIP FLEXION – ISOMETRIC	35					
STRAIGHT LEG RAISE (SLR)	36					
STRAIGHT LEG RAISE (SLR) – ANKLE WEIGHTS	37					
STRAIGHT LEG RAISE (SLR) - ELASTIC BAND	38					
SEATED MARCHING	39					
SEATED MARCHING - ELASTIC BAND	40					
HIP EXTENSION - PRONE	41					
HIP EXTENSION – PRONE – ANKLE WEIGHTS	42					
HIP EXTENSION – PRONE – ELASTIC BAND	43					
HIP EXTENSION – QUADRUPED	44					
HIP ABDUCTION - SUPINE	45					
HIP ABDUCTION - SUPINE – ANKLE WEIGHTS	46					
HIP ABDUCTION – SUPINE - ELASTIC BAND	47					
HIP ABDUCTION / CLAMS– SUPINE - ELASTIC BAND	48					
MODIFIED HIP ABDUCTION – SIDELYING	49					

EXERCISE Lower Extremity - Lying & Seated Strengthening and Range of Motion	EXERCISE NUMBER	PAGE	REPS	SETS	X DAY	HOLD
HIP ABDUCTION – SIDELYING	50					
HIP ABDUCTION – SIDELYING - WEIGHTS	51					
HIP ABDUCTION – SIDELYING - ELASTIC BAND	52					
CLAM SHELLS	53					
SIDELYING CLAM - ELASTIC BAND	54					
HIP ABDUCTION - FIRE HYDRANT - QUADRUPED	55					
HIP ABDUCTION - FIRE HYDRANT – QUADRUPED - ELASTIC BAND	56					
HIP ABDUCTION - SEATED - STRAIGHT LEG	57					
HIP ABDUCTION - SEATED - STRAIGHT LEG – ANKLE WEIGHT	58					
HIP ABDUCTION - SINGLE- SEATED	59					
HIP ABDUCTION - SINGLE- SEATED – ELASTIC BAND	60					
HIP ABDUCTION - BILATERAL- SEATED	61					
HIP ABDUCTION - BILATERAL- SEATED - ELASTIC BAND	62					
HIP ADDUCTION SQUEEZE – SUPINE – KNEES BENT	63					
HIP ADDUCTION SQUEEZE – SUPINE – LEGS STRAIGHT	64					
HIP ADDUCTION - SIDELYING	65					
INTERNAL ROTATION - HEEL SQUEEZE - ISOMETRIC	67					
HIP INTERNAL ROTATION - SUPINE	68					
REVERSE CLAMS - SIDELYING	69					
REVERSE CLAMS - SIDELYING - ELASTIC BAND	70					
HIP INTERNAL ROTATION - SEATED	71					
HIP INTERNAL ROTATION - ELASTIC BAND	72					
HIP EXTERNAL ROTATION - SUPINE	73					

EXERCISE Lower Extremity - Lying & Seated Strengthening and Range of Motion	EXERCISE NUMBER	PAGE	REPS	SETS	X DAY	HOLD
HIP EXTERNAL ROTATION - ELASTIC BAND	74					
HIP ROTATIONS – BILATERAL - SIDELYING	75					
HIP ROTATION - SEATED - BALL and ELASTIC BAND	76					
PRESS – BILATERAL – ELASTIC BAND	77					
PRESS – SINGLE LEG – ELASTIC BAND	78					
HIP HIKE - STANDING	79					
HIP HIKE – KNEELING	80					
GLUTE SETS - PRONE	81					
GLUTE SET - SUPINE	82					
GLUTE SQUEEZE - SITTING	83					
GLUTE SCULPT (MAX/MEDIUS)	84					

EXERCISE Upper Extremity Strengthening and Range of Motion	EXERCISE NUMBER	PAGE	REPS	SETS	X DAY	HOLD
ELBOW FLEXION EXTENSION - SUPINE	1					
ELBOW FLEXION / EXTENSION - GRAVITY ELIMINATED	2					
BICEPS CURLS – ALTERNATING	3					
BICEPS CURL - SELF FIXATION – ELASTIC BAND	4					
SEATED BICEPS CURLS - ALTERNATING	5					
SEATED BICEPS CURLS - BILATERAL	6					
CONCENTRATION CURLS – SITTING	7					
PREACHER CURL ON BALL	8					
BICEPS CURLS	9					
BICEPS CURLS - RADIOBRACHIALIS - HAMMER CURL	10					
BICEPS CURLS - BRACHIALIS	11					
BICEPS CURLS – ROTATE OUTWARD	12					
BICEPS CURLS – ONE ARM - ELASTIC BAND	13					
BICEPS CURLS – BILATERAL - ELASTIC BAND	14					
BICEPS CURLS - RADIOBRACHIALIS - HAMMER CURL – ONE ARM - ELASTIC BAND	15					
BICEPS CURLS - RADIOBRACHIALIS - HAMMER CURL – BILATERAL - ELASTIC BAND	16					
BICEPS CURLS – BRACHIALIS - ONE ARM - ELASTIC BAND	17					
BICEPS CURL – BRACHIALIS – BILATERAL - ELASTIC BAND	18					
TRICEPS - SELF FIXATION - ELASTIC BAND	19					
OVERHEAD TRICEPS - SELF FIXATION –SEATED OR STANDING - ELASTIC BAND	20					
TRICEP EXTENSION – SITTING OR STANDING - WEIGHT	21					
TRICEP EXTENSION – SITTING OR STANDING – BILATERAL - WEIGHT	22					
ELBOW EXTENSION - BALL	23					

EXERCISE Upper Extremity Strengthening and Range of Motion	EXERCISE NUMBER	PAGE	REPS	SETS	X DAY	HOLD
ELBOW EXTENSION - SKULL CRUSHER - BALL	24					
TRICEPS - ELASTIC BAND	25					
TRICEPS - BENT OVER	26					
CHAIR DIPS / PUSH UPS	27					
DIPS OFF CHAIR	28					
PENDULUM SHOULDER FORWARD/BACK	29					
PENDULUM SHOULDER – SIDE TO SIDE	30					
PENDULUM SHOULDER CIRCLES	31					
PENDULUMS - SUPINE	32					
ISOMETRIC FLEXION	33					
SHOULDER FLEXION – SIDELYING	34					
FLEXION – SUPINE - SINGLE OR BILATERAL	35					
FLEXION – SUPINE – SINGLE OR BILATERAL - WEIGHT	36					
FLEXION – SUPINE - DOWEL	37					
FLEXION – SUPINE - DOWEL - Weight	38					
FLEXION - SELF FIXATION – ELASTIC BAND	39					
FLEXION – ELASTIC BAND	40					
FLEXION - STANDING - PALMS DOWN / OVERHAND DOWEL	41					
FLEXION - STANDING - PALMS UP / UNDERHAND DOWEL	42					
FLEXION – PALMS FACING INWARD	43					
FLEXION – PALMS DOWN	44					
V RAISE	45					
V RAISE – WEIGHTS	46					
MILITARY PRESS – DOWEL	47					
MILITARY PRESS - FREE WEIGHTS	48					

EXERCISE Upper Extremity Strengthening and Range of Motion	EXERCISE NUMBER	PAGE	REPS	SETS	X DAY	HOLD
ISOMETRIC EXTENSION	49					
PRONE EXTENSION - EXERCISE BALL	50					
SHOULDER EXTENSION - STANDING	51					
SHOULDER EXTENSION - STANDING - WEIGHTS	52					
EXTENSION – STANDING – DOWEL	53					
EXTENSION - SELF FIXATION - ELASTIC BAND	54					
EXTENSION - ELASTIC BAND	55					
EXTENSION - BILATERAL - ELASTIC BAND	56					
INTERNAL ROTATION – ISOMETRIC	57					
INTERNAL ROTATION - ISOMETRIC- ELEVATED	58					
INTERNAL ROTATION - SIDELYING	59					
INTERNAL ROTATION - ELASTIC BAND	60					
INTERNAL / EXTERNAL ROTATION - STANDING – DOWEL	61					
INTERNAL ROTATION – DOWEL	62					
EXTERNAL ROTATION - ISOMETRIC	63					
EXTERNAL ROTATION - ISOMETRIC – ELEVATED	64					
EXTERNAL ROTATION WITH TOWEL - SIDELYING	65					
EXTERNAL ROTATION – 90/90 - WEIGHTS	66					
EXTERNAL ROTATION - BILATERAL - ELASTIC BAND	67					
EXTERNAL ROTATION - ELASTIC BAND	68					
ADDUCTION – ISOMETRIC	69					
ADDUCTION - ELASTIC BAND	70					
ABDUCTION – ISOMETRIC	71					
HORIZONTAL ABDUCTION - DOWEL	72					

EXERCISE **Upper Extremity Strengthening and Range of Motion**	EXERCISE NUMBER	PAGE	REPS	SETS	X DAY	HOLD
HORIZONTAL ABDUCTION/ADDUCTTION - SUPINE	73					
HORIZONTAL ABDUCTION/ADDUCTTION - SUPINE -WEIGHT	74					
ABDUCTION - SIDELYING	75					
HORIZONTAL ABDUCTION - SIDELYING	76					
ABDUCTION – WEIGHT	77					
ABDUCTION – ELASTIC BAND	78					
HORIZONTAL ABDUCTION – BILATERAL - ELASTIC BAND	79					
90/90 ABDUCTION - WEIGHT	80					
LATERAL RAISES	81					
LATERAL RAISES – LEAN FORWARD	82					
LATERAL RAISES – LEAN FORWARD - ARM ROTATION	83					
FRONTAL RAISE – WEIGHTS	84					
UPRIGHT ROW – WEIGHTS	85					
UPRIGHT ROW – ELASTIC BAND	86					
SHRUGS	87					
SHRUGS - WEIGHTS	88					
SHOULDER ROLLS	89					
SHOULDER ROLLS - WEIGHTS	90					
SCAPULAR RETRACTIONS - BILATERAL	91					
SCAPULAR RETRACTION – SINGLE ARM	92					
ELASTIC BAND SCAPULAR RETRACTIONS WITH MINI SHOULDER EXTENSIONS	93					
PRONE RETRACTION	94					
SCAPULAR PROTRACTION - SUPINE - BILATERAL	95					
SCAPULAR PROTRACTION - SUPINE - WEIGHT	96					

EXERCISE **Upper Extremity** **Strengthening and Range of Motion**	EXERCISE NUMBER	PAGE	REPS	SETS	X DAY	HOLD
SCAPULAR PROTRACTION - SUPINE - ELASTIC BAND	97					
SCAPULAR PROTRACTION / TABLE PLANK	98					
CHEST PRESS – SEATED or STANDING - ELASTIC BAND	99					
CHEST PRESS – BALL, FLOOR or BENCH-WEIGHTS	100					
DOWEL PRESS – STANDING	101					
CHEST PRESS – STANDING or SEATED	102					
BENT OVER ROWS	103					
ROWS – PRONE	104					
ROWS - ELASTIC BAND	105					
WIDE ROWS - ELASTIC BAND	106					
LOW ROW – ELASTIC BAND	107					
HIGH ROW – ELASTIC BAND	108					
FLY'S – FLOOR - WEIGHT	109					
FLY'S – BALL or BENCH – WEIGHT	110					
WALL PUSH UPS	111					
WALL PUSH UP - BALL	112					
WALL PUSH UP - Triceps uneven	113					
WALL PUSH UP - Hands inverted	114					
WALL PUSH UP - Narrow	115					
WALL PUSH UP – Wide	116					
PUSH UPS - BALL	117					
PUSH UP - MODIFIED	118					
PUSH UP	119					
PUSH UP -DIAMOND	120					
PUSH UP – MODIFIED - BOSU - UNSTABLE	121					

EXERCISE Upper Extremity Strengthening and Range of Motion	EXERCISE NUMBER	PAGE	REPS	SETS	X DAY	HOLD
PUSH UP – BOSU - UNSTABLE	122					
PUSH UP – MODIFIED – INVERTED BOSU - UNSTABLE	123					
PUSH UP – INVERTED BOSU - UNSTABLE	124					

EXERCISE Balance / Standing Exercises	EXERCISE NUMBER	PAGE	REPS	SETS	X DAY	HOLD
WIDE BOS DECREASING TO NARROW BOS	1					
NARROW BOS	2					
ARM MOVEMENT	3					
TRUNK ROTATION	4					
EYES SHUTS	5					
HEAD TURNS	6					
READING ALOUD	7					
BALANCE PAD	8					
SPLIT STANCE – SEMI TANDEM	9					
SPLIT STANCE - *Progression*	10					
TANDEM- SHARPENED ROMBERG STANCE	11					
TANDEM STANCE - Progression	12					
SINGLE LEG STANCE (SLS)	13					
SINGLE LEG STANCE (SLS) - *Progression*	14					
SLS – LEG FORWARD	15					
SLS – LEG BACKWARDS	16					
SLS – LEG FORWARD / OPPOSITE ARM UP	17					
SLS – LEG BACKWARDS / OPPOSITE ARM UP	18					
SLS - REACH FORWARD	19					
SLS - REACH TWIST	20					
SINGLE LEG TOE TAP	21					
SINGLE LEG STANCE - CLOCKS	22					
BALL ROLLS - HEEL TOE	23					
BALL ROLLS - LATERAL	24					
SQUAT	25					
SIT TO STAND	26					

EXERCISE Balance / Standing Exercises	EXERCISE NUMBER	PAGE	REPS	SETS	X DAY	HOLD
SQUATS – WALL WITH BALL	27					
SQUATS WITH WEIGHTS	28					
MINI SQUAT - UNSTABLE SUPPORT - FOAM PAD	29					
SQUATS - SINGLE LEG	30					
SIDE TO SIDE WEIGHT SHIFT	31					
FORWARD AND BACKWARDS WEIGHT SHIFTS	32					
SPLIT STANCE WEIGHT SHIFT SIDE TO SIDE	33					
SPLIT STANCE WEIGHT SHIFT FORWARD AND BACKWARDS	34					
WALL FALLS - FORWARD - BALANCE DRILL	35					
WALL FALLS - LATERAL - BALANCE DRILL	36					
WALL FALLS - BACKWARDS - BALANCE DRILL	37					
WALL FALLS - SINGLE LEG - FORWARD - BALANCE DRILL	38					
WALL FALLS - SINGLE LEG - LATERAL - BALANCE DRILL	39					
WALL FALLS - SINGLE LEG - MEDIAL - BALANCE DRILL	40					
WALL FALLS - SINGLE LEG - BACKWARDS - BALANCE DRILL	41					
FALL LATERAL - STEP RECOVERY	42					
FALL FORWARD - STEP RECOVERY	43					
FALL BACKWARD - STEP RECOVERY	44					
TOE TAP ABDUCTION	45					
HIP ABDUCTION - STANDING	46					
HIP EXTENSION – STANDING	47					
HIP FLEXION - STANDING – STRAIGHT LEG RAISE	48					
HIP / KNEE FLEXION - SINGLE LEG	49					
STANDING MARCHING	50					

EXERCISE Balance / Standing Exercises	EXERCISE NUMBER	PAGE	REPS	SETS	X DAY	HOLD
HAMSTRING CURL	51					
TOE RAISES	52					
TOE RAISES IR AND ER	53					
ONE LEGGED TOE RAISE	54					
SINGLE LEG BALANCE FORWARD	55					
SINGLE LEG BALANCE LATERAL	56					
SINGLE LEG BALANCE RETRO	57					
SINGLE LEG STANCE RETROLATERAL	58					
SQUAT	59					
SINGLE LEG SQUAT	60					
LUNGE – STATIC	61					
LUNGE FORWARD/BACKWARD	62					
FOUR CORNER MARCHING IN PLACE	63					
FOUR CORNER MARCHING IN PLACE WITH HEAD TURNS	64					
WALKING ON HEELS FORWARD AND BACKWARDS	65					
WALKING ON TOES FORWARD AND BACKWARDS	66					
TANDEM STANCE AND WALK – FORWARD AND BACKWARDS	67					
RUNNING MAN	68					
HOP STICK - FORWARD	69					
HOP STICK - BACKWARDS	70					
MINI LATERAL LUNGE	71					
SIDE STEPPING	72					
HOP STICK - LATERAL	73					
SINGLE LEG DEAD LIFT	74					

EXERCISE Balance / Standing Exercises	EXERCISE NUMBER	PAGE	REPS	SETS	X DAY	HOLD
CONE TAPS - SINGLE LEG STANCE	75					
CONE TAPS - SINGLE LEG STANCE - UNSTABLE	76					
FIGURE 8 AROUND CONES	77					
FIGURE 8 AROUND CONES – FOOT OR HAND TAP	78					
BALANCE DOUBLE LEG STANCE - WIDE	79					
BALANCE DOUBLE LEG STANCE - NARROW	80					
TANDEM STANCE	81					
TANDEM WALK	82					
SINGLE LEG STANCE - ABDUCTION	83					
SINGLE LEG STANCE - ABDUCTION	84					
SINGLE LEG STANCE – FORWARD KICK	85					
SINGLE LEG STANCE – HAMSTRING CURL	86					
SINGLE LEG SQUAT – LEG FORWARD	87					
SINGLE LEG SQUAT – LEG BACKWARDS	88					
TOE TAP OR HEEL PLACEMENT	89					
PULL UP FOOT TOUCHES ON STEP	90					
ALTERNATING SUSTAINED FOOT TOUCHES ON STEP	91					
STEP UP AND OVER	92					
FORWARD SWING THROUGH STEP	93					
SIDE STEPPING - *REPEAT STEPS 89-93 from a side approach.*	94					

Worksheets

EXERCISE Agility/Reactivity/Speed	EXERCISE NUMBER	PAGE	REPS	SETS	X DAY	HOLD
Four Square Drills	1					
Dots	2					
Ladder Drills	3					
Box Drills	4					
Cones	5					
Hurdles	6					

Myofascial Release

Myofascial release (MFR, self-myofascial release) is an alternative medicine therapy that claims to treat skeletal muscle immobility and pain by relaxing contracted muscles, improving blood and lymphatic circulation, and stimulating the stretch reflex in muscles.

Fascia is a thin, tough, elastic type of connective tissue that wraps most structures within the human body, including muscle. Fascia supports and protects these structures. Osteopathic theory proposes that this soft tissue can become restricted due to psychogenic disease, overuse, trauma, infectious agents, or inactivity, often resulting in pain, muscle tension, and corresponding diminished blood flow. (Wikipedia - *https://en.wikipedia.org/wiki/Myofascial_release*)

Possible Benefits of Myofascial Release

- Muscle relaxation
- Improves muscular and joint range of motion
- Reduces muscle soreness and improves tissue recovery
- Encourages the flow of lymph.
- Improves neuromuscular efficiency.
- Reduces adhesions and scar tissue.
- Releases trigger point (sensitivity and pain) – brings in blood flow and nutrient exchange.
- Maintains normal functional muscular length / Provides optimal length-tension relationship.
- Corrects muscle imbalances

USE

- Roll on foam roller or ball until you find the sore spot or trigger point. When you find this point, stop and rest on it or decrease the range to this particular area and hold for 10-20 seconds.
- Apply pressure to muscle area only. Try not to roll over bones, joints or directly on the spine (you can use a ball over the muscles on the side of the spine).
- Use this as a part of your warmup for particular areas you are exercising that day (for instance the hamstrings, calves and quadricep on leg strengthening day)
- You can use this technique on additional days for trouble areas and can even devote a dedicated session for whole body myofascial release.

Equipment Needed: FOAM ROLLER and/or TEXTURED or SOFT MASSAGE BALL

EXERCISE	EXERCISE NUMBER	NOTES
Myofascial Release		
ANTERIOR CHEST - BALL	1	
ANTERIOR CHEST - FOAM ROLL	2	
LATISSIMUS DORSI – BALL	3	
LATISSIMUS DORSI - FOAM ROLL	4	
TRICEP – FOAM ROLL	5	
OCCIPITAL RELEASE - FOAM ROLL	6	
THORACIC MOBILIZATION – SUPINE - FOAM ROLL	7	
THORACIC MOBILIZATION – STANDING - FOAM ROLL	8	
LUMBAR – STANDING – BALL - can do with foam roll	9	
LUMBAR – SUPINE – FOAM ROLLER	10	
HIP FLEXORS - BALL	11	
HIP FLEXORS – FOAM ROLL	12	
QUADRICEPS – BILATERAL - FOAM ROLL	13	
QUADRICEP – SINGLE - FOAM ROLL	14	
GLUTE /PIRIFORMIS - FOAM ROLL	15	
HIP ADDUCTORS – FOAM ROLL	16	
HAMSTRING – BILATERAL - FOAM ROLL	17	
HAMSTRING – SINGLE – FOAM ROLL	18	
CALVES – BILATERAL - FOAM ROLL	19	
CALVES – SINGLE - FOAM ROLL	20	
ILIOTIBIAL BAND (IT Band) - FOAM ROLL	21	
ILIOTIBIAL BAND (IT Band) - BALL	22	
PLANTAR FASCIA ROLLING – BALL	23	
PLANTAR FASCIA ROLLING - COLD SODA CAN	24	

Myofascial Release

	_____ Reps _____ Sets _____ X Day _____ Hold		_____ Reps _____ Sets _____ X Day _____ Hold
1	Notes:	**2**	Notes:

ANTERIOR CHEST - BALL

Face towards the wall and place small ball at the outside of chest. Bend knees up and down to find the target point and hold.

ANTERIOR CHEST - FOAM ROLL

Lie face down so that a foam roll is under the upper part of your arm and chest. Using your other arm and legs, roll forward and back across this area.

	_____ Reps _____ Sets _____ X Day _____ Hold		_____ Reps _____ Sets _____ X Day _____ Hold
3	Notes:	**4**	Notes:

LATISSIMUS DORSI – BALL

Turn with your target side towards the wall and place small ball on the side under the shoulder. Bend knees up and down to find the target point and hold.

LATISSIMUS DORSI - FOAM ROLL

Lie on your side so that a foam roll is under the upper part of your arm and back. Using your other arm and legs, roll forward and back across this area.

	_____ Reps _____ Sets _____X Day _____Hold		_____ Reps _____ Sets _____X Day _____Hold
5	Notes:	6	Notes:

TRICEP – FOAM ROLL

In a sidelying position, place your tricep on the foam roll. Use the opposite arm and your body to help roll out the arm on the foam roll.

OCCIPITAL RELEASE - FOAM ROLL

Lie on your back and put a foam roll under the back of your head. Turn your head slowly from side to side.

	_____ Reps _____ Sets _____X Day _____Hold		_____ Reps _____ Sets _____X Day _____Hold
7	Notes:	8	Notes:

THORACIC MOBILIZATION – SUPINE - FOAM ROLL

Lie on a foam roller. While supporting your neck, roll up and down your mid-back.

THORACIC MOBILIZATION – STANDING - FOAM ROLL

Stand with a foam roll behind your upper back. Slowly perform mini-squats and allow the foam roller to roll up and down your back for a self-massage.

	_____ Reps _____ Sets _____X Day _____Hold		_____ Reps _____ Sets _____X Day _____Hold
9	Notes:	**10**	Notes:

LUMBAR – STANDING – BALL - can do with foam roll

Place small ball in lower back on the side of the spine. DO NOT roll directly over the spine. Slowly perform mini-squats and allow the ball to roll up and down your back for a self-massage.
*Can use foam roll behind lower back and follow above directions.

LUMBAR – SUPINE – FOAM ROLLER

Lie on a foam roll under the lower back. While supporting your upper body, roll up and down your lower back.

	_____ Reps _____ Sets _____X Day _____Hold		_____ Reps _____ Sets _____X Day _____Hold
11	Notes:	**12**	Notes:

Ball under hip flexor

HIP FLEXORS - BALL

Lie on your stomach and place small ball under hip flexor. Roll up and down ball making small movements and hold on the target muscle.

HIP FLEXORS – FOAM ROLL

Lie on your stomach and place foam roll under both hip flexors. Roll up and down avoiding rolling directly over hip bones.

13	_____ Reps _____ Sets _____ X Day _____ Hold
	Notes:

14	_____ Reps _____ Sets _____ X Day _____ Hold
	Notes:

QUADRICEPS – BILATERAL - FOAM ROLL

Lie face down so that a foam roll is under the top of your thighs. Using your arms propped on your elbows, roll forward and back across this area.

QUADRICEP – SINGLE - FOAM ROLL

Lie face down so that a foam roll is under the top of your target thigh. Cross your other leg over the top of your target leg. Using your arms propped on your elbows, roll forward and back across this area.

15	_____ Reps _____ Sets _____ X Day _____ Hold
	Notes:

16	_____ Reps _____ Sets _____ X Day _____ Hold
	Notes:

GLUTE /PIRIFORMIS - FOAM ROLL

Sit on a foam roll and cross your affected leg on top of your other knee. Lean slightly towards your target side. Using your arms and unaffected leg roll forward and back across your buttock area.

HIP ADDUCTORS – FOAM ROLL

Lie on your stomach supported by arms and lace your inner thigh on the roller. Roll and compress the target thigh muscle.

	_____ Reps _____ Sets _____ X Day _____ Hold		_____ Reps _____ Sets _____ X Day _____ Hold
17	Notes:	18	Notes:

HAMSTRING – BILATERAL - FOAM ROLL

Sit on a foam roll under both thighs. Using your arms, roll forward and back across this area

HAMSTRING – SINGLE – FOAM ROLL

Sit on a foam roll under thigh. Using your arms, roll forward and back across this area.

	_____ Reps _____ Sets _____ X Day _____ Hold		_____ Reps _____ Sets _____ X Day _____ Hold
19	Notes:	20	Notes:

CALVES – BILATERAL - FOAM ROLL

Sit with the foam roll under your both your calves. Lift your body up with your arms and roll forward and back across your calf area. Try turning toes in and out to access the inside and outside of calf areas. Do not roll in the crease of your knee.

CALVES – SINGLE - FOAM ROLL

Sit with the foam roll under your target calf and cross your other leg on top. Lift your body up with your arms and roll forward and back across your calf area. Do not roll in the crease of your knee.

_____ Reps _____ Sets _____ X Day _____ Hold		_____ Reps _____ Sets _____ X Day _____ Hold
21	Notes:	**22**	Notes:

ILIOTIBIAL BAND (IT Band) - FOAM ROLL

Lie on your side with a foam roll under your bottom thigh. Use your arms and unaffected leg and then roll up and down the foam roll along the outside of your thigh.

ILIOTIBIAL BAND (IT Band) - BALL

Lie on your side or sit in chair. Hold small ball and move along the outside of the thigh. Hold on the target muscle.

_____ Reps _____ Sets _____ X Day _____ Hold		_____ Reps _____ Sets _____ X Day _____ Hold
23	Notes:	**24**	Notes:

PLANTAR FASCIA ROLLING – BALL

Sit and place ball under foot. Roll plantar fascia over ball back and forth.

PLANTAR FASCIA ROLLING - COLD SODA CAN

Sit and place cold soda can under foot. Roll plantar fascia over can back and forth.

Flexibility (Stretching)

Range of motion within a joint across various planes of motion that can be increased with stretching. This is needed to prevent decreased range of motion in a joint. Joint mobility can be inhibited by body habitués, genetics, connective tissue elasticity, skin that surrounds the joint, or the joint itself.

Some of the benefits of stretching: *(ACE Personal Training Manual)*	• Increased physical efficiency and performance. • Decreased risk of injury by decreasing resistance in various tissues. • Increased blood supply and nutrients to joint structures. • Improved nutrient exchange by increasing the quantity and decreasing the thickness of synovial fluid in the joint. • Increased neuromuscular coordination. • Improved muscular balance and postural awareness. • Reduced muscular tension. *(Bryant & Daniel, Ace Personal Training Manual, 2003, pg 306-307)*
Things to remember when stretching	• It is always better to stretch a warm muscle (*see Warm up and Cool down*) when the tissue temperature is above normal. Think of putting an elastic band in the freezer compared to heating it before stretching. Which do you think will get a better stretch? • Static stretching is best for the type for beginning athletes. Static stretching is a slow, gradual lengthening of the connective tissue (tendon, muscles and ligaments) through a full range of motion to the point of discomfort – not pain. This stretch should be held for at least 30 seconds, but no longer than two minutes. • Dynamic stretching consists of controlled leg and arm swings that take you to the limits of your range of motion. This type of stretching is appropriate to perform part of a warmup and/or cool down. • Ballistic stretching is a rapid, bouncing movement that may be appropriate in some sports. The problem is that there is also a high-risk factor for injury and should only be done with a professional's guidance. • Again, always remember to warm up before stretching. Repeat all stretches 2-3 times and hold for 15-30 seconds up to 60 seconds) unless otherwise indicated. • Some evidence shows that static stretching may be more beneficial at the end of the exercise program when there is more certainty that the muscles have warmed up. • Dynamic stretching may be more beneficial at the beginning of the exercise program as part of your warmup. This can also be done at the end as part of the cool down.

Flexibility (Stretching)

EXERCISE Flexibility (Stretching)	EXERCISE NUMBER	NOTES
INVERSION	1	
EVERSION	2	
ANTERIOR TIBIALIS	3	
PLANTARFLEXION	4	
DORSIFLEXION - STRAP	5	
DORSIFLEXION - FLOOR ASSISTED	6	
STANDING CALF STRETCH - GASTROC	7	
STANDING CALF STRETCH - GASTROC – HAND ON KNEE	8	
GASTROCNEMIUS STAIR STRETCH	9	
STANDING CALF STRETCH - SOLEUS	10	
HAMSTRING STRETCH – TOWEL, BAND, STRAP or BELT	11	
HAMSTRING STRETCH – TOWEL, BAND, STRAP or BELT	12	
HAMSTRING STRETCH - TABLE, BED OR COUCH	13	
HAMSTRING / KNEE EXTENSION STRETCH - SEATED	14	
HAMSTRING STRETCH - STANDING	15	
TOE TOUCH – STANDING - NARROW or WIDE BOS	16	
HEEL SLIDES - SELF ASSISTED	17	
HEEL SLIDES - LONG SIT ASSISTED - TOWEL, BAND, STRAP or BELT	18	
HEEL SLIDES - SUPINE	19	
KNEE BENDS - EXERCISE BALL	20	
KNEE FLEXION – SELF ASSISTED - PRONE	21	
KNEE FLEXION – BELT ASSISTED - PRONE	22	
HEEL SLIDES - SELF ASSISTED	23	
HEEL SLIDES - SEATED	24	
KNEE FLEXION – SCOOT FORWARD - SEATED	25	

Flexibility (Stretching)

EXERCISE Flexibility (Stretching)	EXERCISE NUMBER	NOTES
KNEE FLEXION – STAIR OR STEP	26	
PIRIFORMIS STRETCH	27	
PIRIFORMIS STRETCH - EXERCISE BALL	28	
PIRIFORMIS STRETCH - LONG SIT	29	
PIRIFORMIS STRETCH – STANDING	30	
HIP FLEXOR STRETCH - SIDE OF BALL or CHAIR	31	
HIP FLEXOR STRETCH - STANDING	32	
HIP FLEXOR STRETCH - HALF KNEEL	33	
RUNNER'S STRETCH - MODIFIED	34	
HIP FLEXOR STRETCH – SUPINE	35	
HIP FLEXOR STRETCH – SUPINE - 2	36	
QUAD STRETCH - SIDELYING	37	
QUAD STRETCH - STANDING	38	
KNEE FALL OUT STRETCH or FROG STRETCH	39	
BUTTERFLY STRETCH	40	
HIP ADDUCTOR STRECH – KNEELING	41	
HIP ADDUCTOR STRECH - STANDING	42	
HIP EXTERNAL ROTATION STRETCH - SUPINE	43	
HIP INTERNAL ROTATION STRETCH - SEATED	44	
IT BAND STRETCH - STANDING	45	
IT BAND STRETCH -- SIDELYING	46	
NECK ROTATION and SIDE BENDS	47	
NECK FLEXION AND EXTENSION	48	
TRUNK FLEXION - SEATED	49	
LOW BACK STRETCH - SEATED	50	
LOW BACK STRETCH – STANDING - STRAIGHT & LATERAL	51	
LOW BACK STRETCH – RAIL OR DOORKNOB	52	

EXERCISE Flexibility (Stretching)	EXERCISE NUMBER	NOTES
PRAYER STRETCH and LATERAL	53	
PRAYER STRETCH - EXERCISE BALL	54	
CAT AND CAMEL	55	
KNEE TO CHEST STRETCH - SINGLE and BILATERAL	56	
PRONE ON ELBOWS	57	
PRESS UPS	58	
TRUNK ROTATION STRETCH – SINGLE LEG	59	
LOWER TRUNK ROTATIONS – BILATERAL	60	
TRUNK ROTATION - SEATED	61	
TRUNK ROTATION - STANDING or SEATED – DOWEL	62	
LATERAL TRUNK STRETCH - SINGLE, SEATED or STANDING	63	
LATERAL TRUNK STRETCH - BILATERAL SEATED or STANDING	64	
FLEXION - SUPINE - DOWEL	65	
WALL WALK	66	
FLEXION - TABLE SLIDE	67	
FLEXION - TABLE SLIDE - BALL	68	
EXTERNAL ROTATION - SUPINE – DOWEL *INTERNAL ROTATION ON OPPOSITE ARM*	69	
EXTERNAL ROTATION - 90-90 - DOWEL	70	
EXTERNAL ROTATION – SEATED – DOWEL *INTERNAL ROTATION ON OPPOSITE ARM*	71	
EXTERNAL ROTATION – STANDING – DOWEL *INTERNAL ROTATION ON OPPOSITE ARM*	72	
ABDUCTION - TABLE SLIDE - BALL	75	
ABDUCTION WITH DOWEL	76	
LYING DOWN EXTENSION - TABLE or BED	77	
WAND EXTENSION - STANDING	78	
CHEST STRETCH – SEATED, STANDING, or SUPINE	79	

Flexibility (Stretching)

EXERCISE Flexibility (Stretching)	EXERCISE NUMBER	NOTES
TRICEP STRETCH - STRAP or TOWEL	82	
POSTERIOR SHOULDER/DELTOID RELEASE	83	
POSTERIOR CAPSULE STRETCH	84	

Stretching / Range of Motion (ROM)

Inversion

_____ Reps _____ Sets _____X Day _____Hold

1 | Notes:

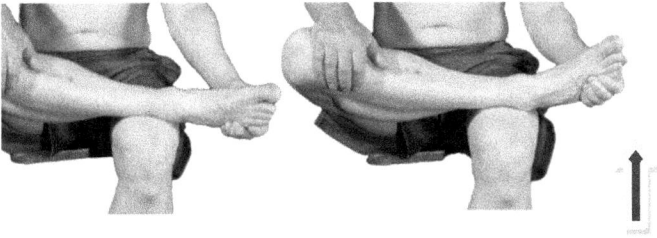

INVERSION

Sit and cross your legs so that the target leg is on top. Hold your foot and pull upwards until a stretch is felt along the side of your ankle.

Eversion

_____ Reps _____ Sets _____X Day _____Hold

2 | Notes:

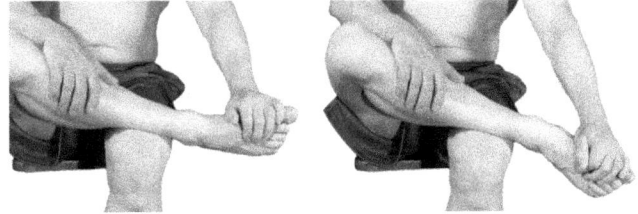

EVERSION

Sit and cross your legs so that the target leg is on top. Hold your foot and push downward until a stretch is felt along the inner side of your ankle.

Anterior Tibialis (Ant Tib)

_____ Reps _____ Sets _____X Day _____Hold

3 | Notes:

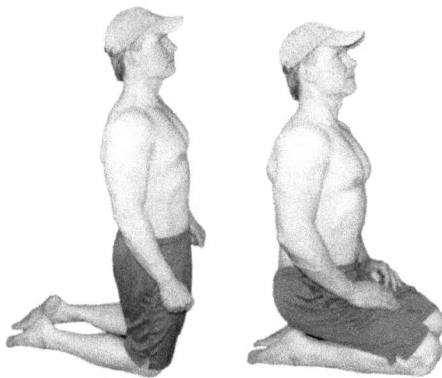

ANTERIOR TIBIALIS

Kneel upright and slowly sit back onto legs forcing heels down towards floor. Sit back until stretch is felt.

Plantarflexion (PF) _DF not shown_

_____ Reps _____ Sets _____X Day _____Hold

4 | Notes:

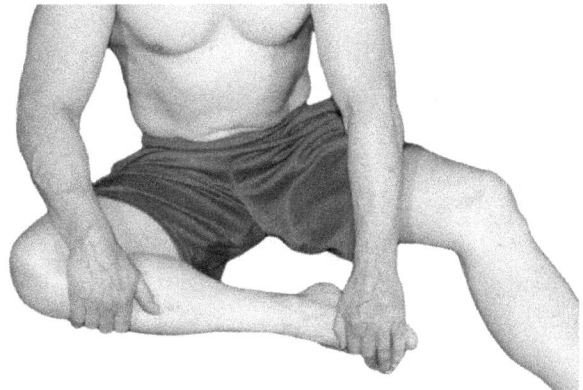

PLANTARFLEXION

Sit and place your affected foot on a firm surface. Use one hand bend the ankle downward as shown.

DORSIFLEXION – _Not shown_
Sit and place your affected foot on a firm surface. Use one hand under foot to push up towards shin (see #5 for movement)

Dorsiflexion (DF)

5	_____ Reps _____ Sets _____ X Day _____ Hold
	Notes:

DORSIFLEXION - STRAP

Sit with heel on floor and leg straight. Place belt/strap on forefoot and pull back until stretch is felt.

6	_____ Reps _____ Sets _____ X Day _____ Hold
	Notes:

DORSIFLEXION - FLOOR ASSISTED

Sit and slide your foot back towards under the chair until a stretch is felt at the ankle.

Gastroc/Soleus

7	_____ Reps _____ Sets _____ X Day _____ Hold
	Notes:

Target Leg

STANDING CALF STRETCH - GASTROC

Stand in front of a wall, chair, or other sturdy object. Step forward with one foot and maintain your toes on both feet to be pointed straight forward. Keep the leg behind you with a straight knee during the stretch. Lean forward as you allow your front knee to bend until a stretch is felt along the back of your leg. Move closer or further away from the wall to control the stretch of the back leg.

8	_____ Reps _____ Sets _____ X Day _____ Hold
	Notes:

Target Leg

STANDING CALF STRETCH - GASTROC – HAND ON KNEE

Step forward with one foot and place hand on thigh. Maintain your toes on both feet to be pointed straight forward. Keep the leg behind you with a straight knee during the stretch. Lean forward as you allow your front knee to bend until a stretch is felt along the back of your leg. You can adjust the bend of the front knee to control the stretch.

	_____ Reps _____ Sets _____X Day _____Hold		_____ Reps _____ Sets _____X Day _____Hold
9	Notes:	10	Notes:

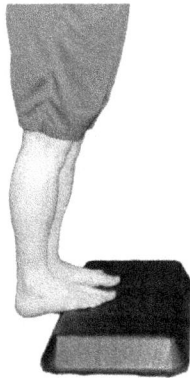

GASTROCNEMIUS STAIR STRETCH

Stand with the middle of your foot on the edge of the stairs while holding onto the railing. Slowly drop heels off until you feel a stretch in the back of your legs keeping your knees straight.

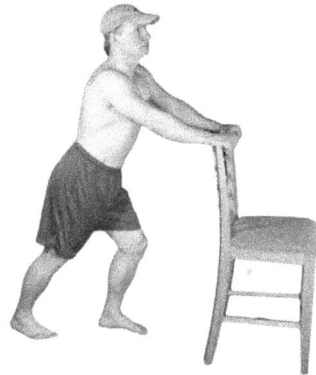

STANDING CALF STRETCH - SOLEUS

Stand in front of a wall, chair or other sturdy object. Step forward with one foot and maintain your toes on both feet to be pointed straight forward. Keep the leg behind you with a slightly bent knee during the stretch. Lean forward towards the wall and support yourself with your arms as you allow your front knee to bend until a gentle stretch is felt along the back of your leg. *Move closer or further away from the wall to control the stretch of the back leg. You can also adjust the bend of the front knee to control the stretch.

Hamstring / Knee Extension

	_____ Reps _____ Sets _____X Day _____Hold		_____ Reps _____ Sets _____X Day _____Hold
11	Notes:	12	Notes:

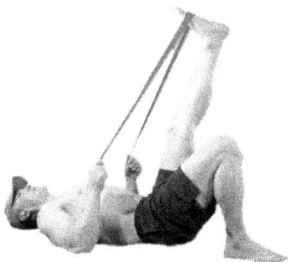

HAMSTRING STRETCH – TOWEL, BAND, STRAP or BELT

Lie down on your back and hook a towel/strap under your foot and draw up your leg until a stretch is felt under your leg/calf area. Keep your knee in a straightened position during the stretch. To increase stretch move strap to forefoot and flex foot.

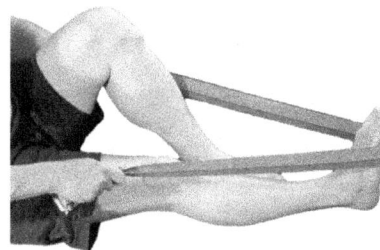

HAMSTRING STRETCH – TOWEL, BAND, STRAP or BELT

While pushing down on thigh above knee cap with opposite hand, pull on towel/ strap to lift heel from floor. Keep thigh flat. To increase stretch move strap to forefoot and flex foot and/or lean forward at the hip.

Flexibility (Stretching)

	_____ Reps _____ Sets _____X Day _____Hold		_____ Reps _____ Sets _____X Day _____Hold
13	Notes:	**14**	Notes:

HAMSTRING STRETCH - TABLE, BED OR COUCH

Sit on a raised flat surface where you can prop your target leg up on it such as a treatment table, couch or bed. While keeping your knee straight, slowly lean forward and reach your hands towards your foot until a gentle stretch is felt along the back of your knee/thigh. Hold and then return to starting position and repeat. Allow gravity to stretch your knee towards a more straightened position.
* Can use strap, towel or belt around forefoot as in #12

HAMSTRING / KNEE EXTENSION STRETCH - SEATED

Sit and tighten your top thigh muscle to press the back of your knee downward towards the ground. You should feel a gentle stretch in the back of your knee.

* To increase stretch put strap to forefoot, flex foot and lean forward at the hip.

	_____ Reps _____ Sets _____X Day _____Hold		_____ Reps _____ Sets _____X Day _____Hold
15	Notes:	**16**	Notes:

HAMSTRING STRETCH - STANDING

Stand and rest your foot on a stool/box/step with your knee straight. Gently lean forward at the hips until a stretch is felt behind your knee/thigh. Keep your back straight. *To increase stretch, flex your foot at the ankle, and/or put strap to forefoot and flex foot. If on stair, you can put foot on 2nd or 3rd step.

TOE TOUCH – STANDING - NARROW or WIDE BOS

Stand and bend forward at waist keep legs straight and reach for toes. Can perform with either narrow or wide base of support.

Knee Flexion

_____ Reps _____ Sets _____X Day _____Hold		_____ Reps _____ Sets _____X Day _____Hold
17	Notes:	**18** Notes:

HEEL SLIDES - SELF ASSISTED

Lie on your back with knees straight and slide the target heel towards your buttock as you bend your knee. Use the unaffected leg to assist the bending. Hold a gentle stretch in this position and then return to original position.

HEEL SLIDES - LONG SIT ASSISTED - TOWEL, BAND, STRAP or BELT

Sit with legs straight. Can place a small hand towel under your heel to help slide. Loop a band around your foot and pull your knee into a bend position as your foot slides towards your buttock. Hold a gentle stretch and then return back to original position.

_____ Reps _____ Sets _____X Day _____Hold		_____ Reps _____ Sets _____X Day _____Hold
19	Notes:	**20** Notes:

HEEL SLIDES - SUPINE

Lie on your back with knees straight and slide the target heel towards your buttock as you bend your knee. Hold a gentle stretch in this position and then return to original position.

KNEE BENDS - EXERCISE BALL

Lie on your back and place your heels on an exercise ball. Roll it closer to your buttocks as your knees and hips bend as shown. Hold and then return to original position. *If you have limited range in one knee, use the other leg to help increase range of motion.

Flexibility (Stretching)

_____ Reps _____ Sets _____ X Day _____ Hold		_____ Reps _____ Sets _____ X Day _____ Hold
21	Notes:	**22** Notes:

KNEE FLEXION – SELF ASSISTED - PRONE

Lie face down and bend your target knee with the assistance of your unaffected leg.

KNEE FLEXION – BELT ASSISTED - PRONE

Lie face down with a strap looped around your target side ankle or foot. Use the belt to pull the knee into a bent position allowing for a stretch.

_____ Reps _____ Sets _____ X Day _____ Hold		_____ Reps _____ Sets _____ X Day _____ Hold
23	Notes:	**24** Notes:

HEEL SLIDES - SELF ASSISTED

It and slide your heel towards your buttock with the assist of the unaffected leg. Hold a gentle stretch and then return foot forward to original position.

HEEL SLIDES - SEATED – can use towel or paper under foot to help slide

Sit and place your feet on the floor (can put target foot on a towel or paper to help slide if needed). Slowly slide your foot closer towards you. Hold a gentle stretch and then return foot forward to original position.

	_____ Reps _____ Sets _____X Day _____Hold
25	**Notes:**

Plant foot.
Scoot hips
forward.

KNEE FLEXION – SCOOT FORWARD - SEATED

Sit and slide your foot back to a bent knee position. Keep your foot planted on the ground and scoot forward until a stretch is felt at the knee. Hold the stretch and then scoot back to original position.

	_____ Reps _____ Sets _____X Day _____Hold
26	**Notes:**

KNEE FLEXION – STAIR OR STEP

Place target foot on stool or step with bent knee. Gently bend forward keeping heel on step. Hold the stretch and then return to original position.

Piriformis

	_____ Reps _____ Sets _____X Day _____Hold
27	**Notes:**

PIRIFORMIS STRETCH

Lie on your back with both knees bent. Cross your target leg on the other knee. Hold your unaffected thigh and pull it up towards your chest until a stretch is felt in the buttock.

	_____ Reps _____ Sets _____X Day _____Hold
28	**Notes:**

PIRIFORMIS STRETCH - EXERCISE BALL

Lie on your back with one foot placed on the ball. Cross your other leg over the knee of the leg on the ball and gently roll the ball back towards your chest until a stretch is felt in the buttock.

	_____ Reps _____ Sets _____X Day _____Hold		_____ Reps _____ Sets _____X Day _____Hold
29	Notes:	**30**	Notes:

PIRIFORMIS STRETCH - LONG SIT

Sit with one knee straight and the other bent and placed over the opposite knee. Gentle turn your body towards the bend knee side.

PIRIFORMIS STRETCH – STANDING

Stand with unaffected leg crossed in front of target side. Lean forward reaching for foot on target side until stretch is felt in the buttock.

Hip Flexors

	_____ Reps _____ Sets _____X Day _____Hold		_____ Reps _____ Sets _____X Day _____Hold
31	Notes:	**32**	Notes:

HIP FLEXOR STRETCH - SIDE OF BALL or CHAIR

Sit on edge of chair or ball. Bend your front knee (unaffected side) and lean forward until a stretch is felt along the front of the target hip.

HIP FLEXOR STRETCH - STANDING

Stand and bend one knee forward (unaffected side) and the other in back. Stand up straight leaning slightly backward until a stretch is felt along the front of the target hip.

_____ Reps _____ Sets _____ X Day _____ Hold

33	Notes:

HIP FLEXOR STRETCH - HALF KNEEL – with or without pad under knee

Begin in a half-kneeling position (you may want to use a pad or pillow for cushion). Bend your front knee (unaffected side) and lean forward until a stretch is felt along the front of the target hip.

_____ Reps _____ Sets _____ X Day _____ Hold

34	Notes:

RUNNER'S STRETCH - MODIFIED

Stretch target leg in back and bend other knee in front. Bend your front knee (unaffected side) and lean forward until a stretch is felt along the front of the target hip.

_____ Reps _____ Sets _____ X Day _____ Hold

35	Notes:

HIP FLEXOR STRETCH – SUPINE

Lie on a table, high bed or matt and let the affected leg lower towards the floor until a stretch is felt along the front of your thigh.

_____ Reps _____ Sets _____ X Day _____ Hold

36	Notes:

HIP FLEXOR STRETCH – SUPINE

Lie on a table, high bed or matt and let the affected leg lower towards the floor until a stretch is felt along the front of your thigh. At the same time, grasp your opposite knee and pull it towards your chest.

Quadriceps (Quad)

	_____ Reps _____ Sets _____ X Day _____ Hold		_____ Reps _____ Sets _____ X Day _____ Hold
37	Notes:	**38**	Notes:

QUAD STRETCH - SIDELYING

Lie on your side and reach back holding the top of your foot with bent knee until a stretch is felt.

QUAD STRETCH - STANDING

Stand straight up and bend your knee in back holding your ankle/foot. Gently pull your knee/thigh back in alignment with the standing leg.

Adductor

	_____ Reps _____ Sets _____ X Day _____ Hold		_____ Reps _____ Sets _____ X Day _____ Hold
39	Notes:	**40**	Notes:

One Leg

Both Legs

KNEE FALL OUT STRETCH or FROG STRETCH

Lie on your back with one knee bent. Slowly lower your knee to the side as you stretch the inner thigh/hip area. Frog Stretch: Let both knees fall to the side at the same time.

BUTTERFLY STRETCH

Sit on the floor or mat and bend your knees placing the bottom of your feet together. Slowly let your knees lower towards the floor until a stretch is felt at your inner thighs.

	_____ Reps _____ Sets _____X Day _____Hold
41	Notes:

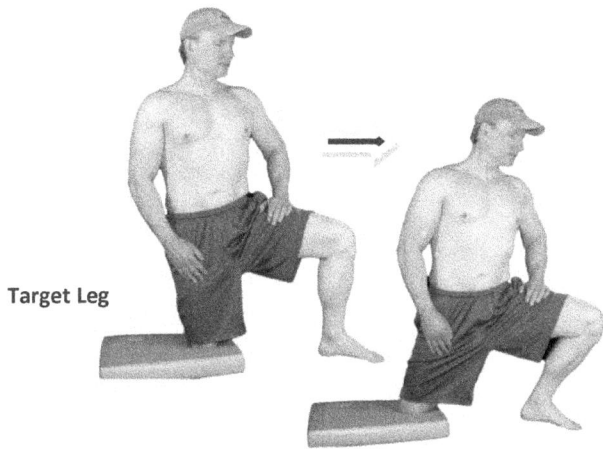

HIP ADDUCTOR STRECH – KNEELING

Kneel down on your target side knee. Place the opposite leg directly out to the side. Lean towards the side as you bend the knee for a stretch to the inner thigh of the target leg.

	_____ Reps _____ Sets _____X Day _____Hold
42	Notes:

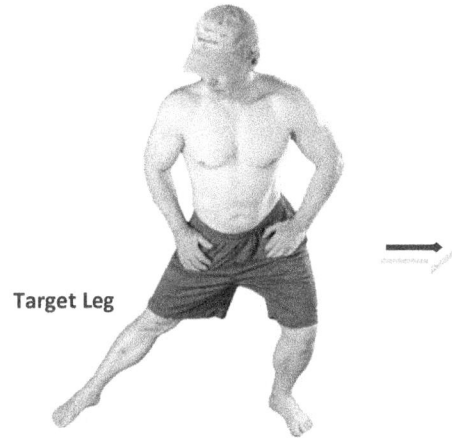

HIP ADDUCTOR STRECH - STANDING

Stand with feet spread wide apart. Slowly bend your knee to allow for a gentle stretch of the opposite leg. Maintain a straight knee on the target leg the entire time. You should feel a stretch on the inner thigh.

External Rotation / Internal Rotation

	_____ Reps _____ Sets _____X Day _____Hold
43	Notes:

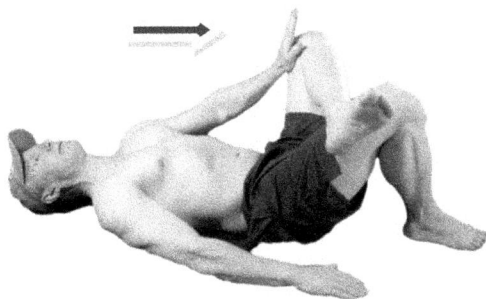

HIP EXTERNAL ROTATION STRETCH - SUPINE

Lie on your back with your leg crossed over your knee. Use your hand and push the crossed knee away from you.

	_____ Reps _____ Sets _____X Day _____Hold
44	Notes:

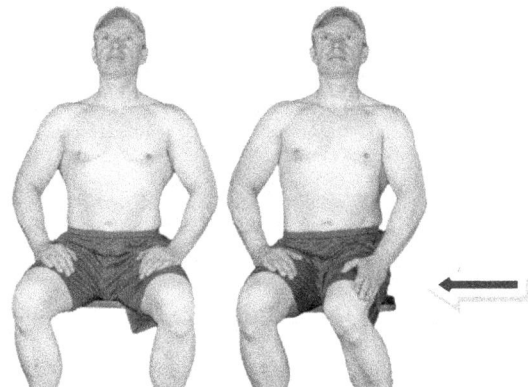

HIP INTERNAL ROTATION STRETCH - SEATED

Sit on a chair with your legs spread apart and feet planted on the ground. Use your hand to draw your knee inward as shown.

Iliotibial Band (IT Band)

_____ Reps _____ Sets _____ X Day _____ Hold		_____ Reps _____ Sets _____ X Day _____ Hold
45	Notes:	**46**	Notes:

IT BAND STRETCH - STANDING

Stand and cross the target leg behind your unaffected leg. Lean forward and towards the unaffected side while using your arm for balance support.

IT BAND STRETCH -- SIDELYING

Lie on bed or couch on unaffected side with target side towards ceiling. Bend lower leg for support. Allow upper leg to drop over side of bed. Keep knee straight and point toe towards floor. May need to roll upper hip backwards in order to feel stretch on side of hip/thigh/knee.

NECK

_____ Reps _____ Sets _____ X Day _____ Hold		_____ Reps _____ Sets _____ X Day _____ Hold
47	Notes:	**48**	Notes:

NECK ROTATION and SIDE BENDS

SIDE BENDS: (_Top_) Tilt your head as if you are trying to touch your ear to your shoulder. For extra stretch gently use your hand to increase range and hold.
ROTATION: (_Bottom_) Turn your head to the side as if looking over your shoulder. For an extra stretch gently use your hand on your chin to increase range and hold.

NECK FLEXION AND EXTENSION

EXTENSION: Look up as if you are looking at the sky moving your neck only.
FLEXION: Look down as if you are looking at the floor. For an extra stretch gently put both hands behind your head to move chin towards the chest and hold.

BACK

	_____ Reps _____ Sets _____X Day _____Hold	_____ Reps _____ Sets _____X Day _____Hold
49	Notes:	**50** Notes:

TRUNK FLEXION - SEATED

Sit and cross your arms over your chest. Slowly curl your back forward in order to round your upper back.

LOW BACK STRETCH - SEATED

Sit and slowly bend forward reaching your hands for the floor. Bend your trunk and head forward and down.

	_____ Reps _____ Sets _____X Day _____Hold	_____ Reps _____ Sets _____X Day _____Hold
51	Notes:	**52** Notes:

LOW BACK STRETCH – STANDING - STRAIGHT & LATERAL

Stand in front of a table / chair or other surface and bend forward at the waist. Support yourself with your hands on a surface.

Reach to the side for a lateral bend (see #53)

LOW BACK STRETCH – RAIL OR DOORKNOB

Hold onto doorknob, rail or other unmovable surface and pull while moving hips back and hold.

_____ Reps _____ Sets _____X Day _____Hold		_____ Reps _____ Sets _____X Day _____Hold	
53	Notes:	**54**	Notes:

Lateral

Straight

PRAYER STRETCH and LATERAL

STRAIGHT: Start on your hands and knees. Slowly lower your buttocks towards your feet until a stretch is felt along your back and or buttocks.

LATERAL: Start on your hands and knees. Slowly lower your buttocks towards your feet. Lower your chest towards the floor as you reach out towards the side.

PRAYER STRETCH - EXERCISE BALL

Kneel with an exercise ball in front of you. Slowly lean forward and roll the ball forward until a stretch is felt.

*Can do lateral movement as in #53

_____ Reps _____ Sets _____X Day _____Hold		_____ Reps _____ Sets _____X Day _____Hold	
55	Notes:	**56**	Notes:

CAT AND CAMEL

Start on your hands and knees. Raise up your back and arch it towards the ceiling (cat). Return to a lowered position and arch your back the opposite direction (camel).

Both Legs

One Leg

KNEE TO CHEST STRETCH - SINGLE and BILATERAL

BILATERAL: Lie on your back and hold your knees while pulling up towards your chest and hold.
SINGLE: Lie on your back and hold your knee while pulling up towards your chest and hold. Opposite leg can be straight or bent.

Trunk Extension

	_____ Reps _____ Sets _____ X Day _____ Hold		_____ Reps _____ Sets _____ X Day _____ Hold
57	Notes:	**58**	Notes:

PRONE ON ELBOWS

Lie on your stomach. Slowly press up and prop yourself up on your elbows. Keep hips on floor/mat.

PRESS UPS

Lie on your stomach. Slowly press up and arch your back using your arms. Keep hips on floor/mat.

Trunk Rotation

	_____ Reps _____ Sets _____ X Day _____ Hold		_____ Reps _____ Sets _____ X Day _____ Hold
59	Notes:	**60**	Notes:

TRUNK ROTATION STRETCH – SINGLE LEG

Lie on your back with arms to the sides. Bend one knee and then raise it up and across your body. Allow your trunk to rotate for a gentle stretch to the spine. Hold and then repeat.

LOWER TRUNK ROTATIONS – BILATERAL

Lie on your back with your knees bent and gently move your knees side-to-side.

Flexibility (Stretching)

_____ Reps _____ Sets _____X Day _____Hold	_____ Reps _____ Sets _____X Day _____Hold
61 Notes:	**62** Notes:

TRUNK ROTATION - SEATED

Sit up as tall with erect posture. Rotate in one direction, using your hand to press against the opposite thigh to aide in further rotation. Exhale to increase the rotation and stretch. Return to the starting position, maintain an upright posture -repeat in the opposite direction.

TRUNK ROTATION - STANDING or SEATED – DOWEL

Stand or sit holding dowel in hands. Slowly rotate trunk in one direction and then in the opposite direction.

Lateral

_____ Reps _____ Sets _____X Day _____Hold	_____ Reps _____ Sets _____X Day _____Hold
63 Notes:	**64** Notes:

LATERAL TRUNK STRETCH - SINGLE SEATED or STANDING

Raise your arm and bend to the opposite side for a stretch. Hold and repeat with opposite arm.

LATERAL TRUNK STRETCH - BILATERAL SEATED or STANDING

Clasp hands together and raise arms over head. Bend to one side. Hold and repeat in opposite direction.

Shoulder Flexion

	_____ Reps _____ Sets _____X Day _____Hold		_____ Reps _____ Sets _____X Day _____Hold
65	Notes:	**66**	Notes:

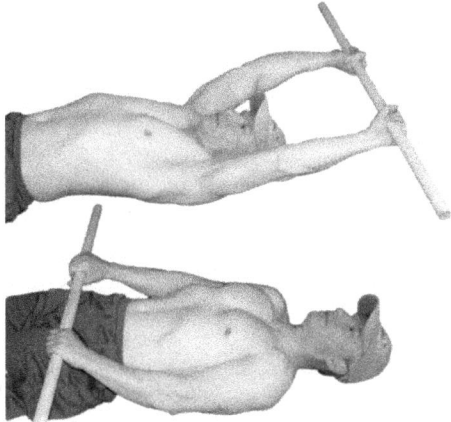

FLEXION - SUPINE - DOWEL

Lie on your back and hold a dowel/cane. Slowly raise the dowel overhead.

*If you have a weak or injured arm, you can use your unaffected arm to assist with the movement.

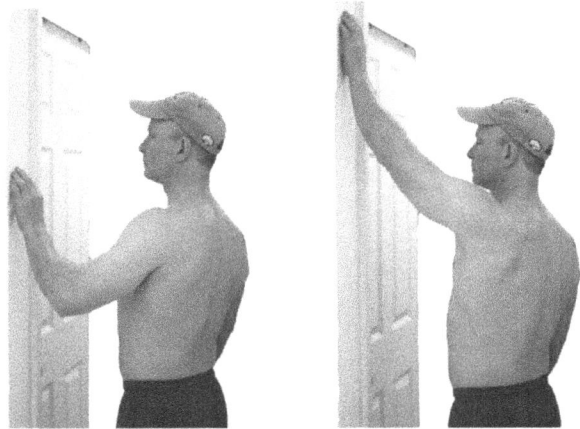

WALL WALK

Place your target hand on the wall with the palm facing the wall. Walk your fingers up the wall towards overhead. Slide or walk your hand back down the wall to the starting position.

	_____ Reps _____ Sets _____X Day _____Hold		_____ Reps _____ Sets _____X Day _____Hold
67	Notes:	**68**	Notes:

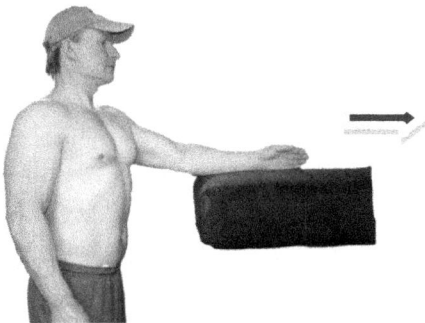

FLEXION - TABLE SLIDE

Sit or stand and rest your target arm on a table and gently slide it forward and then back.

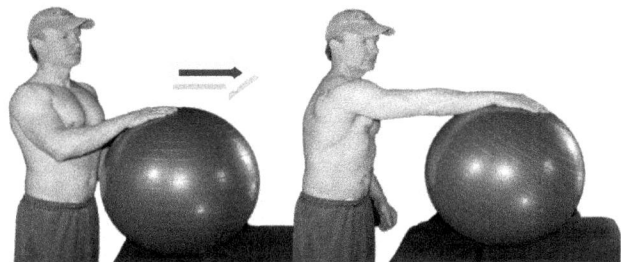

FLEXION - TABLE SLIDE - BALL

Stand and rest your target arm on top of a ball on a table. Gently roll the ball forward and then back.

Shoulder External Rotation (ER)

	_____ Reps _____ Sets _____ X Day _____ Hold		_____ Reps _____ Sets _____ X Day _____ Hold
69	**Notes:**	**70**	**Notes:**

Starting Position

EXTERNAL ROTATION - SUPINE – DOWEL
INTERNAL ROTATION ON OPPOSITE ARM

Lie on your back holding a dowel/cane with both hands. On the target side, maintain approx. 90-degree bend at the elbow with your arm approximately 30-45 degrees away from your side. Use your other arm to push the dowel/cane to rotate the affected arm back into a stretch. Hold and then return to starting position. Repeat

EXTERNAL ROTATION - 90-90 - DOWEL

Lie on your back and hold a dowel with your elbows out to the side and rested down. Roll your arms back towards overhead until a stretch is felt. Keep elbows bent at a 90-degree angle.

	_____ Reps _____ Sets _____ X Day _____ Hold		_____ Reps _____ Sets _____ X Day _____ Hold
71	**Notes:**	**72**	**Notes:**

EXTERNAL ROTATION – SEATED – DOWEL
INTERNAL ROTATION ON OPPOSITE ARM

Using the unaffected arm, push the dowel into the hand of the target arm. Keep the arm at a 90-degree angle and push until a stretch is felt. Hold and repeat.

EXTERNAL ROTATION – STANDING – DOWEL
INTERNAL ROTATION ON OPPOSITE ARM

Using the unaffected arm, push the dowel into the hand of the target arm. Keep the arm at a 90-degree angle and push until a stretch is felt. Hold and repeat.

Shoulder Internal Rotation (IR) - *also see #69, 71, 72*

_____ Reps _____ Sets _____X Day _____Hold		_____ Reps _____ Sets _____X Day _____Hold	
73	Notes:	**74**	Notes:

INTERNAL ROTATION – TOWEL OR STRAP

Hold one end of the towel in front and with the target arm behind your back. Gently pull up your target arm behind your back with the assist of a towel.

INTERNAL ROTATION – DOWEL

Hold a dowel/cane behind your back. Slowly pull the target arm towards the center of your back.

Shoulder Abduction

_____ Reps _____ Sets _____X Day _____Hold		_____ Reps _____ Sets _____X Day _____Hold	
75	Notes:	**76**	Notes:

ABDUCTION - TABLE SLIDE - BALL

Stand and rest your target arm on top of a ball on a table and gently roll it to the side and back.

ABDUCTION WITH DOWEL

Hold a dowel/cane in front. Slowly push the dowel of the unaffected arm towards the target arm upward and to the side.

Shoulder Extension

	_____ Reps _____ Sets _____X Day _____Hold		_____ Reps _____ Sets _____X Day _____Hold
77	**Notes:**	**78**	**Notes:**

LYING DOWN EXTENSION - TABLE or BED

Lie on your back and gently let target arm drop off table or bed.

WAND EXTENSION - STANDING

Stand and hold a dowel/cane. Use the unaffected arm to help push the target arm back. The elbow should remain straight the entire time.

Chest/Pec Stretch

	_____ Reps _____ Sets _____X Day _____Hold		_____ Reps _____ Sets _____X Day _____Hold
79	**Notes:**	**80**	**Notes:**

CHEST STRETCH – SEATED, STANDING, or SUPINE

TOP: Bend arms at a 90-degree angle. Move elbows back until feeling a stretch in front of shoulders/chest.

BOTTOM: Clasp hands in back of head. Move elbows back until feeling a stretch in front of shoulders/chest.

CHEST STRETCH - STEP THROUGH

Stand with arms in doorway at a 90-degree angle. Step through until you feel a stretch through the chest and hold. Keep shoulders down and back. Take another step to increase stretch.

Triceps

_____ Reps _____ Sets _____ X Day _____ Hold	_____ Reps _____ Sets _____ X Day _____ Hold
81 Notes:	**82** Notes:

TRICEP STRETCH

With your target elbow bent and shoulder raised, use your other hand and gently push your target elbow back towards overhead until a stretch is felt.

TRICEP STRETCH - STRAP or TOWEL

Hold strap of target arm with your hand above your head. Use the other hand to pull downward on the strap, allowing the elbow to bend until a stretch is in the back of the arm.

Posterior Capsule

_____ Reps _____ Sets _____ X Day _____ Hold	_____ Reps _____ Sets _____ X Day _____ Hold
83 Notes:	**84** Notes:

POSTERIOR SHOULDER/DELTOID RELEASE

Bring your target arm across your body. Use the opposite hand to grasp the back of your shoulder and further pull the arm. Hold.

POSTERIOR CAPSULE STRETCH

Lie on your side and grasp the elbow of the arm closest to the floor. Gently pull it upward and across the front of your body.

Core / Stability Training

Core strengthening is the foundation of all the other exercises that follow, especially balance. Core training is not only an important step in conditioning, but also helps other issues, including neurological, orthopedic, weight, or overall weakness

The core includes muscles of the thoraco-lumbar spine (trunk), cervical spine., erector spinae, abdomen, pelvis, shoulder/scapulae, and your lower lats.

Static core functionality is the ability of one's core to align the skeleton to resist a force that does not change. The core is used to stabilize the thorax and the pelvis during dynamic movement. The nature of dynamic movement must consider our skeletal structure (as a lever) in addition to the force of external resistance and consequently incorporates a vastly different complex of muscles and joints versus a static position.

The core is traditionally assumed to originate most full-body functional movement, including most sports. In addition, the core determines to a large part a person's posture. In all, human anatomy is built to take force upon the bones and direct autonomic force, through various joints, in the desired direction. The core muscles align the spine, ribs, and pelvis of a person to resist a specific force, whether static or dynamic.
(Wikipedia: *https://en.wikipedia.org/wiki/Core_(anatomy)*)

These muscles work as stabilizers for the entire body. Core training is simply doing specific exercises to develop and strengthen these stabilizer muscles. If any of these core muscles are weakened, it could result in lower back pain or a protruding waistline. Keeping these core muscles strong can do wonders for your posture and help give you more strength in other exercises like running and walking.
(Bodybuilding.com - *https://www.bodybuilding.com/fun/mielke12.htm*)

There is a saying 'form follows function'. This is especially true with core stability and how it affects your balance. Gravity influences all movement, so effective core training must be done against gravity. The rectus abdominus muscle that you are isolating with those crunches flexes the spine/abs only when you are lying on your back or returning the torso to an upright position from hyperextension in standing. "In the upright position, flexion is controlled by eccentric contraction of the back extensors as the lower the weight of the torso in the same direction as gravity". (*Bryant & Green, 2003, p. 84*)

Being able to engage the core with not only your balance exercises but also arm and leg exercises will help prevent injury.

Step 1: First learn to brace the abdomen *(see pictures 1 and 2 on next page)* Think of this as trying to either brace for a punch to the stomach or trying to put on a tight pair of pants (not just sucking in your stomach)

Step 2: After getting a good feel for bracing, try doing a pelvic tilt *(see pictures 3 and 4 on next page)* and then progress to bridging *(see picture 5)*

Step 3: These two basic movements should be done while you progress your abdominal and core training, continuing through the balance section, and to some extent with arm and leg strengthening.

*** When doing floor work, such as crunches, make sure you are on a soft surface, such as a mat, Bosu, stability ball, etc. Pushing your back into a hard surface, such as a wood floor, can do more damage than good to the spine.

*** Breathe – Never hold your breath.

EXERCISE Core / Stability	EXERCISE NUMBER	NOTES
ABDOMINAL BRACING TRAINING	1	
ABDOMINAL BRACING - SUPINE	2	
PELVIC TILT - SUPINE	3	
PELVIC TILT - KNEELING	4	
BRIDGING	5	
BRIDGE - BOSU	6	
BRIDGING WITH PILLOW SQUEEZE	7	
BRIDGING WITH PILLOW SQUEEZE - BOSU	8	
BRACE SUPINE MARCHING / BRIDGE LEG UP	9	
BRIDGE LEG UP - BOSU -	10	
SINGLE LEG BRIDGE	11	
BRIDGE SINGLE LEG - BOSU	12	
BRIDGING CROSSED LEG	13	
BRIDGING CROSSED LEG – BOSU	14	
BRIDGING CROSSED LEG - ARMS UP	15	
BRIDGING CROSSED LEG - ARMS UP - BOSU	16	
BRIDGE - ELASTIC BAND	17	
BRIDGING - ABDUCTION - ELASTIC BAND	18	
FLOOR BRIDGE - EXERCISE BALL	19	
FLOOR BRIDGE ALTERNATE LEG LIFT - EXERCISE BALL	20	
BRIDGE UPPER BACK - EXERCISE BALL	21	
BRIDGE UPPER BACK - SINGLE LEG - EXERCISE BALL	22	
QUADRUPED ALTERNATE ARM	23	
QUADRUPED ALTERNATE LEG	24	
QUADRUPED ALTERNATE ARM AND LEG	25	
BIRD DOG ELBOW TOUCHES	26	

EXERCISE	EXERCISE NUMBER	NOTES
Core / Stability		
PRONE BALL	27	
PRONE BALL - ALTERNATE ARM	28	
PRONE BALL - ALTERNATE LEG	29	
PRONE BALL - ALTERNATE ARM AND LEG	30	
MODIFIED PLANK	31	
MODIFIED PLANK - ALTERNATE LEG	32	
FULL PLANK	33	
PLANK - ALTERNATE ARMS	34	
PLANK - ALTERNATE LEGS	35	
PLANK - EXERCISE BALL	36	
PRONE ON ELBOWS	37	
PRESS UPS	38	
SKYDIVER	39	
PRONE SUPERMAN - BOSU	40	
TRUNK EXTENSION - BOSU	41	
TRUNK EXTENSION - HANDS CROSSED IN FRONT - BOSU	43	
SUPERMAN - ARMS BACK- EXERCISE BALL	44	
SUPERMAN – BOTH ARMS IN FRONT - EXERCISE BALL	45	
SUPERMAN – ONE ARM FORWARD / ONE ARM BACK - EXERCISE BALL	46	
LATERAL PLANK MODIFIED	47	
LATERAL PLANK MODIFIED- BOSU	48	
LATERAL PLANK - 1 KNEE 1 FOOT	49	
LATERAL PLANK - 1 KNEE 1 FOOT – BOSU	50	
LATERAL PLANK	51	
LATERAL PLANK - BOSU	52	

EXERCISE Core / Stability	EXERCISE NUMBER	NOTES
LEAN BACK	53	
LEAN BACK - BOSU	54	
LEAN BACK WITH ARMS OUT	55	
LEAN BACK WITH ARMS OUT - BOSU	56	
LEAN BACK WITH TWIST	57	
LEAN BACK WITH TWIST – BOSU	58	
CRUNCHY FROG	59	
SEATED BIKE - FORWARD AND BACKWARDS	60	
CRUNCH – ARMS OUT	61	
CRUNCH – ARMS OUT - BOSU	62	
CRUNCH – ARMS IN BACK OF HEAD	63	
CRUNCH – ARMS IN BACK OF HEAD - BOSU	64	
OBLIQUE CRUNCH	65	
OBLIQUE CRUNCH - BOSU	66	
90 DEGREE CRUNCH	67	
BALL CRUNCH – Can put legs on seat of chair	68	
CURL UPS – ARMS ON LEGS - EXERCISE BALL	69	
CURL UPS- ARMS CROSSED IN FRONT - EXERCISE BALL	70	
CURL UPS – ARMS BEHIND HEAD - EXERCISE BALL	71	
SUPINE CRUNCH TOUCH - EXERCISE BALL	72	
LOWER ABDOMINAL CRUNCH – WITH or WITHOUT BALL	73	
HIGH MARCH CRUNCH	74	
STANDING SIDE CRUNCH	75	
STANDING BIKE CRUNCH	76	

Core/Abdominal

Abdominal Bracing – Pelvic Tilt

	_____ Reps _____ Sets _____X Day _____Hold
1	Notes:

ABDOMINAL BRACING TRAINING

Press your fingertips into your relaxed abdomen lateral of your navel. Tighten and brace your abdomen so that the muscles push your fingertips away from the center of your body. Hold, relax and repeat.
Think of this as trying to either brace for a punch to the stomach or trying to put on a tight pair of pants (not just sucking in your stomach)

	_____ Reps _____ Sets _____X Day _____Hold
2	Notes:

Starting Position

ABDOMINAL BRACING - SUPINE

Lie on your back. Tighten your stomach muscles as you draw your navel down towards the floor.

Think of this as trying to either brace for a punch to the stomach or trying to put on a tight pair of pants (not just sucking in your stomach)

	_____ Reps _____ Sets _____X Day _____Hold
3	Notes:

Starting

Position

PELVIC TILT - SUPINE

Lie on your back with your knees bent. Next, arch your low back and then flatten it repeatedly (bracing as above). Your pelvis should tilt forward and back during the movement. Move through a comfortable range of motion.

	_____ Reps _____ Sets _____X Day _____Hold
4	Notes:

Starting

Position

PELVIC TILT - KNEELING

Kneel on the floor (you can kneel on a pillow or pad if needed). Arch your lower back and then flatten it repeatedly (bracing as above). Your pelvis should tilt forward and back during the movement. Move through a comfortable range of motion.

Bridging

	_____ Reps _____ Sets _____X Day _____Hold		_____ Reps _____ Sets _____X Day _____Hold
5	**Notes:**	**6**	**Notes:**

Starting

Position

BRIDGING

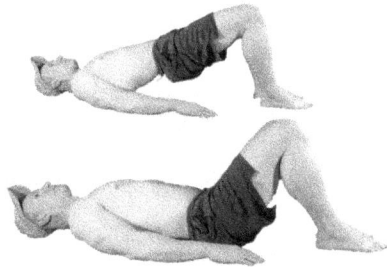

Lie on your back. Tighten your lower abdominals (as with abdominal bracing), squeeze your buttocks and then raise your buttocks off the floor/bed. Hold and then lower yourself slowly and repeat. Brace the stomach muscles to keep your spine from moving, trying to keep the pelvis level the entire time.

Starting

Position

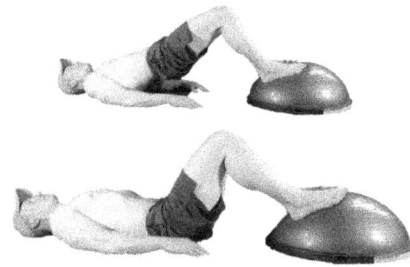

BRIDGE - BOSU – Can use foam pad, stair step or box

Lie on your back with your feet planted on top of the Bosu and knees bent. Lift up your buttocks as shown. Hold and then lower yourself slowly and repeat.
Brace the stomach muscles to keep your spine from moving, trying to keep the pelvis level the entire time.

	_____ Reps _____ Sets _____X Day _____Hold		_____ Reps _____ Sets _____X Day _____Hold
7	**Notes:**	**8**	**Notes:**

Starting

Position

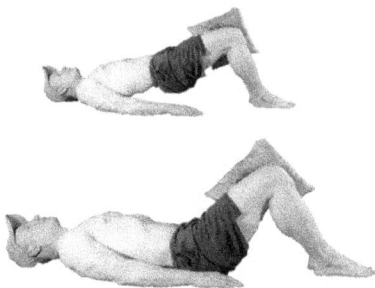

BRIDGING WITH PILLOW SQUEEZE - Use pillow, ball or rolled towel between knees

Lie on your back and place a pillow, towel roll or ball between your knees and squeeze. Hold this and then tighten your lower abdominals, squeeze your buttocks and raise your buttocks off the floor/bed. Brace the stomach muscles to keep your spine from moving, trying to keep the pelvis level.

Starting

Position

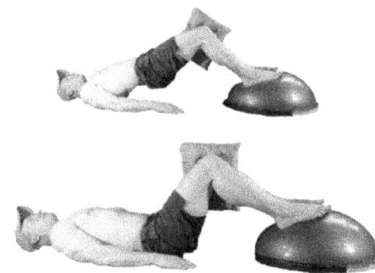

BRIDGING WITH PILLOW SQUEEZE - BOSU - Can use foam pad, stair step or box

Lie on your back with your feet planted on top of the Bosu and knees bent. Place a pillow, towel roll or ball between your knees and squeeze. Lift up your buttocks as shown. Hold and then lower yourself slowly and repeat. Brace the stomach muscles to keep your spine from moving, trying to keep the pelvis level.

	_____ Reps _____ Sets _____ X Day _____ Hold
9	**Notes:**

BRACE SUPINE MARCHING / BRIDGE LEG UP

Lie on your back with your knees bent, slowly lift up one foot a few inches and then set it back down. Perform on your other leg. Brace the stomach muscles to keep your spine from moving, trying to keep the pelvis level the entire time.
*To increase challenge, go into bridge position as with #5, then continue march – can bring leg higher to advance

	_____ Reps _____ Sets _____ X Day _____ Hold
10	**Notes:**

BRIDGE LEG UP - BOSU - Can use foam pad, stair step or box

Lie on your back with your feet planted on top of the Bosu and knees bent. Slowly lift up one foot a few inches and then set it back down. Next, perform on your other leg. Brace the stomach muscles to keep your spine from moving, trying to keep the pelvis level the entire time. *To increase challenge, go into bridge position as with #6, then continue march – can bring leg higher to advance

	_____ Reps _____ Sets _____ X Day _____ Hold
11	**Notes:**

SINGLE LEG BRIDGE

Lie on your back, raise your buttocks off the floor/bed into a bridge position. Straighten a leg so that only one leg is supporting your body. Then, return that leg back to the ground and change to the other side. Brace the stomach muscles to keep your spine from moving, trying to keep the pelvis level the entire time.

	_____ Reps _____ Sets _____ X Day _____ Hold
12	**Notes:**

BRIDGE SINGLE LEG - BOSU - can use foam pad, stair step or box

Lie on your back with your feet planted on top of the Bosu and knees bent, lift up your buttocks and then straighten one knee in the air. Return that leg back to the ground and change to the other side. Brace the stomach muscles to keep your spine from moving, trying to keep the pelvis level the entire time.

	_____ Reps _____ Sets _____X Day _____Hold		_____ Reps _____ Sets _____X Day _____Hold
13	Notes:	14	Notes:

Starting
Position

BRIDGING CROSSED LEG

Lie on your back, cross your leg. Tighten your lower abdomen, squeeze your buttocks and raise your buttocks off the floor/bed. Brace the stomach muscles to keep your spine from moving, trying to keep the pelvis level the entire time.

Starting Position

BRIDGING CROSSED LEG – BOSU - can use foam pad, stair step or box

Lie on your back with your feet planted on top of the Bosu cross your leg. Tighten your lower abdomen, squeeze your buttocks and raise your buttocks. Brace the stomach muscles to keep your spine from moving, trying to keep the pelvis level the entire time.

	_____ Reps _____ Sets _____X Day _____Hold		_____ Reps _____ Sets _____X Day _____Hold
15	Notes:	16	Notes:

Starting
Position

BRIDGING CROSSED LEG - ARMS UP

Lie on your back, cross your leg and put your hands together as shown. Next, tighten your lower abdomen, squeeze your buttocks and raise your buttocks off the floor/bed. Brace the stomach muscles to keep your spine from moving, trying to keep the pelvis level the entire time.

BRIDGING CROSSED LEG - ARMS UP - BOSU - can use foam pad, stair step or box

Lie on your back with your feet planted on top of the Bosu and hands together and leg crossed. Tighten your lower abdomen, squeeze your buttocks and raise your buttocks. Brace the stomach muscles to keep your spine from moving, trying to keep the pelvis level.

	_____ Reps _____ Sets _____X Day _____Hold
17	Notes:

BRIDGE - ELASTIC BAND

Lie on your back, hold an elastic band down around your waist for resistance. Tighten your lower abdomen, squeeze your buttocks and then raise your buttocks off the floor/bed. Brace the stomach muscles to keep your spine from moving, trying to keep the pelvis level the entire time.

	_____ Reps _____ Sets _____X Day _____Hold
18	Notes:

BRIDGING - ABDUCTION - ELASTIC BAND – can be done with feet on BOSU, foam, stair step or box

Lie on your back, place an elastic band around your knees and pull your knees apart. Hold this and then tighten your lower abdomen, squeeze your buttocks and raise your buttocks off the floor/bed. Brace the stomach muscles to keep your spine from moving, trying to keep the pelvis level the entire time.

	_____ Reps _____ Sets _____X Day _____Hold
19	Notes:

FLOOR BRIDGE - EXERCISE BALL

Lie on the floor, place an exercise ball under your lower legs and then raise up your buttocks. Hold and repeat. Brace the stomach muscles to keep your spine from moving, trying to keep the pelvis level the entire time.

	_____ Reps _____ Sets _____X Day _____Hold
20	Notes:

FLOOR BRIDGE ALTERNATE LEG LIFT - EXERCISE BALL

Lie on the floor, place an exercise ball under your lower legs and then raise up your buttocks. While holding this position raise up a leg off the ball towards the ceiling then lower back to the ball and alternate to lift the other leg. Brace the stomach muscles to keep your spine from moving, trying to keep the pelvis level.

_____ Reps _____ Sets _____ X Day _____ Hold

21 | **Notes:**

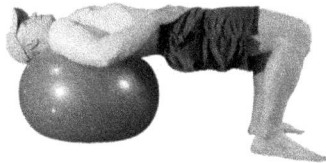

BRIDGE UPPER BACK - EXERCISE BALL

Start in a seated position on the ball and slowly walk your feet forward so that the ball is on your upper back. Keep your buttocks and pelvis up off the ball and straight with your thighs. Brace the stomach muscles to keep your spine from moving, trying to keep the pelvis level the entire time.
*To increase the challenge, you can do a supine march or perform some arm exercises, such as Fly's or Chest Presses (*See Upper Extremity exercises*)

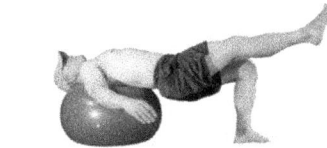

_____ Reps _____ Sets _____ X Day _____ Hold

22 | **Notes:**

Starting

Position

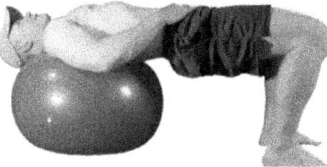

BRIDGE UPPER BACK - SINGLE LEG - EXERCISE BALL

Start in a seated position on the ball and slowly walk your feet forward so that the ball is on your upper back. Keep your buttocks and pelvis up off the ball and straight with your thighs. Raise up one leg so that you straighten your knee in the air. Return it back to the floor and then switch to raise up the other side. Brace the stomach muscles to keep your spine from moving, trying to keep the pelvis level the entire time.

Quadruped

_____ Reps _____ Sets _____ X Day _____ Hold

23 | **Notes:**

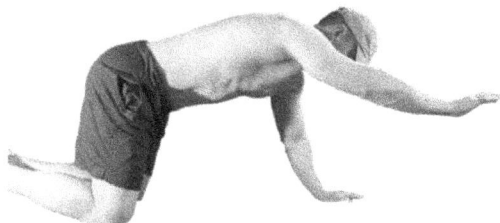

QUADRUPED ALTERNATE ARM

While in a crawling position, slowly raise up an arm out in front of you.

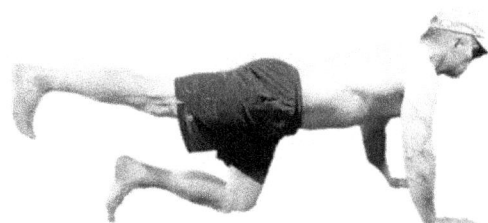

_____ Reps _____ Sets _____ X Day _____ Hold

24 | **Notes:**

QUADRUPED ALTERNATE LEG

While in a crawling position, slowly draw your leg back behind you as you straighten your knee. Either repeat on same side or alternate.

	_____ Reps _____ Sets _____X Day _____Hold		_____ Reps _____ Sets _____X Day _____Hold
25	Notes:	**26**	Notes:

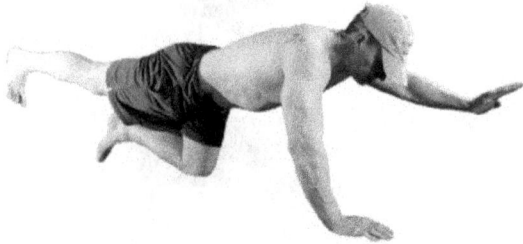

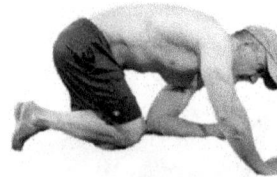

Touch your elbow to your opposite knee

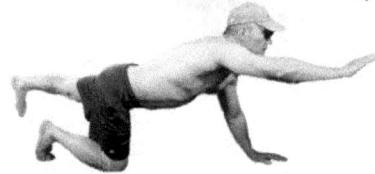

Starting Position

QUADRUPED ALTERNATE ARM AND LEG

While in a crawling position, brace at your abdominals and then slowly lift a leg and opposite arm upwards. Maintain a level and stable pelvis and spine the entire time. Either repeat on same side or alternate.

BIRD DOG ELBOW TOUCHES

While in a crawling position, slowly lift your leg and opposite arm upwards. When returning your arm and leg down, do not touch the floor but instead touch your elbow to your opposite knee and lift and straighten them again. Then set them down on the floor. Either repeat on same side or alternate.

	_____ Reps _____ Sets _____X Day _____Hold		_____ Reps _____ Sets _____X Day _____Hold
27	Notes:	**28**	Notes:

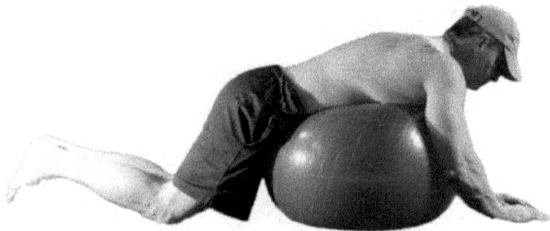

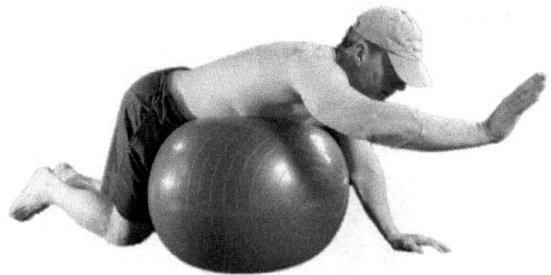

PRONE BALL

Lie face down over a ball, support your self with your feet and hands.

PRONE BALL - ALTERNATE ARM

Lie face down over a ball, support your self with your feet and hands. Next, slowly raise up one arm. Return arm back to floor and then raise up the other arm. Keep alternating arms.

	_____ Reps _____ Sets _____ X Day _____ Hold		_____ Reps _____ Sets _____ X Day _____ Hold
29	Notes:	**30**	Notes:

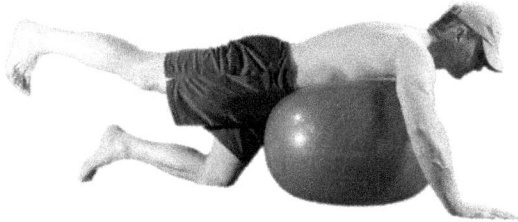

PRONE BALL - ALTERNATE LEG

Lie face down over a ball, support yourself with your arms and legs. Next slowly raise up a leg. Return leg back to floor and then raise up the other leg.

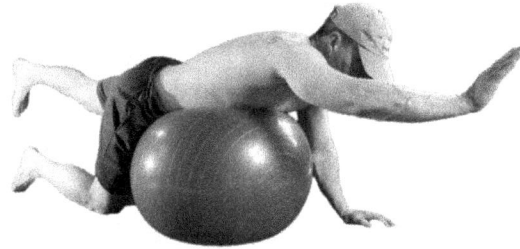

PRONE BALL - ALTERNATE ARM AND LEG

Lie face down over a ball, support yourself with your feet and hands. Next, slowly raise up one arm and opposite leg. Return arm and leg back to floor and then raise up the opposite arm/leg.

Plank

	_____ Reps _____ Sets _____ X Day _____ Hold		_____ Reps _____ Sets _____ X Day _____ Hold
31	Notes:	**32**	Notes:

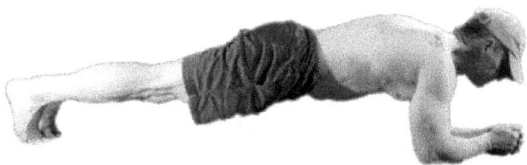

MODIFIED PLANK

Lie face down, lift your body up on your elbows and toes. Try and maintain a straight spine the entire time. Do not allow your low back sag downward.

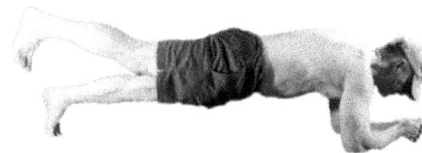

Starting

Position

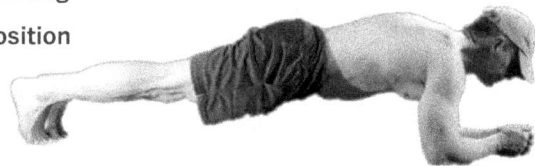

MODIFIED PLANK - ALTERNATE LEG

Lie face down, lift your body up on your elbows and toes. Next, lift one leg off the ground and then set it back down. Then repeat on the other leg. Try and maintain a straight spine the entire time.

	_____ Reps _____ Sets _____X Day _____Hold
33	Notes:

FULL PLANK

Lie face down, lift your body up on your elbows and toes. Straighten your arms in full elbow extension and hold in full plank position. Do not let your back arch down. Try and maintain a straight spine the entire time.

	_____ Reps _____ Sets _____X Day _____Hold
34	Notes:

PLANK - ALTERNATE ARMS

Hold a plank position as previous (#33). Raise one arm out in front of you as shown. Return to the starting position and then raise your other arm out in front of you and repeat.
Try and maintain a straight spine the entire time.

	_____ Reps _____ Sets _____X Day _____Hold
35	Notes:

PLANK - ALTERNATE LEGS

Hold a plank position as previous (#33). Raise one leg off the floor as shown. Return to the starting position and then raise your other leg and repeat. Try and maintain a straight spine the entire time.

	_____ Reps _____ Sets _____X Day _____Hold
36	Notes:

PLANK - EXERCISE BALL

While kneeling on the floor with an exercise ball in front of you, place your elbows and hands on the ball and lift your body up. Try and maintain a straight spine. Do not allow your hips or pelvis on either side to drop.

Back Extension

_____ Reps _____ Sets _____X Day _____Hold		_____ Reps _____ Sets _____X Day _____Hold
37	Notes:	**38**	Notes:

PRONE ON ELBOWS

Lie face down, slowly press up and prop yourself up on your elbows.

PRESS UPS

Lie face down, slowly press up and arch your back using your arms.

_____ Reps _____ Sets _____X Day _____Hold		_____ Reps _____ Sets _____X Day _____Hold
39	Notes:	**40**	Notes:

SKYDIVER

Lie face down with arms by your side. Next, lift your upper body, lower legs, thighs, and arms off the ground at the same time as shown. You can place a pillow under your stomach/hips for comfort.

PRONE SUPERMAN - BOSU

Lie face down over the Bosu. Slowly raise your arms and legs upward off the ground. Then lower slowly back to the ground.

_____ Reps	_____ Sets	_____ X Day	_____ Hold

41

Notes:

Starting

Position

TRUNK EXTENSION - BOSU

Lie face down with your upper body on a Bosu and slowly raise your head and chest upwards as shown.
Your arms can be behind your back or alongside your body.

_____ Reps	_____ Sets	_____ X Day	_____ Hold

42

Notes:

Starting
Position

TRUNK EXTENSION - HANDS BEHIND HEAD - BOSU

Lie face down with your upper body on a Bosu. Touch the back of your head with both hands and slowly raise your head and chest upwards.

_____ Reps	_____ Sets	_____ X Day	_____ Hold

43

Notes:

Starting

Position

TRUNK EXTENSION - HANDS CROSSED IN FRONT - BOSU

While lying face down with your upper body on a Bosu, slowly raise your head and chest upwards.
Keep your arms crossed on your chest as you perform.

_____ Reps	_____ Sets	_____ X Day	_____ Hold

44

Notes:

SUPERMAN - ARMS BACK- EXERCISE BALL

Start in a kneeling position with an exercise ball in front of you. Roll forward so that you are face down on the ball with your feet on the ground and your stomach on the ball. Hold up your head and chest so that a straight line exists between your feet and head. Also bring your arms back along side of your body and hold this position.

_____ Reps _____ Sets _____ X Day _____ Hold		_____ Reps _____ Sets _____ X Day _____ Hold
45	Notes:	**46**	Notes:

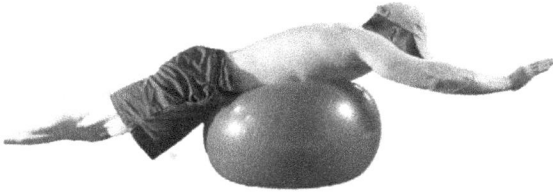

SUPERMAN – BOTH ARMS IN FRONT - EXERCISE BALL

Start in a kneeling position with an exercise ball in front of you. Next, roll forward so that you are face down on the ball with your feet on the ground and your stomach on the ball. Hold up your head and chest so that a straight line exists between your feet and head. Also bring your arms up and forward out in front of you and hold this position.

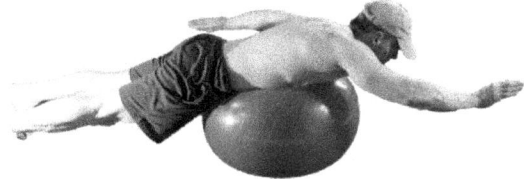

SUPERMAN – ONE ARM FORWARD / ONE ARM BACK - EXERCISE BALL

Start in a kneeling position with an exercise ball in front of you. Next, roll forward so that you are face down on the ball with your feet on the ground and your stomach on the ball. Hold up your head and chest so that a straight line exists between your feet and head. Raise one arm up and out in front of you as you bring the other arm back and along side your body as in a swimming motion.

Lateral Plank

_____ Reps _____ Sets _____ X Day _____ Hold		_____ Reps _____ Sets _____ X Day _____ Hold
47	Notes:	**48**	Notes:

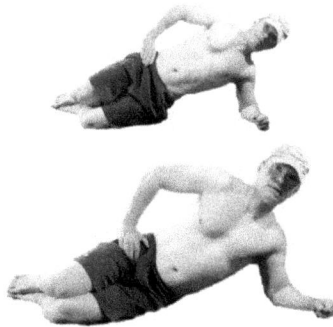

Starting
Position

LATERAL PLANK MODIFIED

Lie on your side with your knees bent, lift your body up on your elbow and knees. Try and maintain a straight spine.

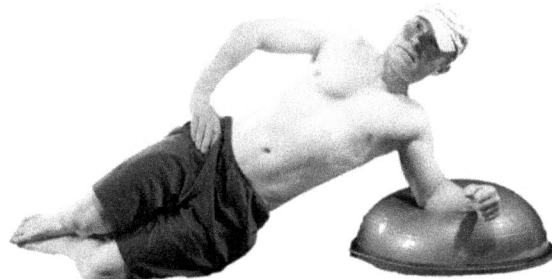

LATERAL PLANK MODIFIED- BOSU- can be anything unstable

Lie on your side with your knees bent and your elbow on the Bosu, lift your body up on your elbow and knees. Try and maintain a straight spine.

	_____ Reps _____ Sets _____X Day _____Hold
49	**Notes:**

LATERAL PLANK - 1 KNEE 1 FOOT

Lie on your side with bottom knee bent and top knee straight. Lift your body up on your elbow and knee on one side and foot on the other side. Try and maintain a straight spine.

	_____ Reps _____ Sets _____X Day _____Hold
50	**Notes:**

LATERAL PLANK - 1 KNEE 1 FOOT – BOSU- Can be anything unstable

Lie on your side with elbow on Bosu with bottom knee bent and the top knee straight. Lift your body up on your elbow and knee on one side and foot on the other side. Try and maintain a straight spine.

	_____ Reps _____ Sets _____X Day _____Hold
51	**Notes:**

Starting

Position

LATERAL PLANK

Lie on your side with both legs straight and lift your body up on your elbow and feet. Try and maintain a straight spine.

	_____ Reps _____ Sets _____X Day _____Hold
52	**Notes:**

LATERAL PLANK - BOSU - Can be anything unstable

Lie on your side with your elbow on the Bosu and both legs straight. Lift your body up on your elbow and feet. Try and maintain a straight spine.

Backward Lean

	_____ Reps _____ Sets _____X Day _____Hold		_____ Reps _____ Sets _____X Day _____Hold
53	Notes:	**54**	Notes:

Starting
Position

LEAN BACK

Start in an upright seated position with knees bent. Hold onto thighs and lean back keeping spine as straight as possible.

Starting
Position

LEAN BACK - BOSU

Start in an upright seated position on Bosu with knees bent. Hold onto thighs or Bosu and lean back keeping spine as straight as possible.

	_____ Reps _____ Sets _____X Day _____Hold		_____ Reps _____ Sets _____X Day _____Hold
55	Notes:	**56**	Notes:

Starting
Position

LEAN BACK WITH ARMS OUT

Start in an upright seated position with knees bent. Hold arms straight out or overhead, brace core and lean back keeping spine as straight as possible

Starting
Position

LEAN BACK WITH ARMS OUT - BOSU

Start in an upright seated position on Bosu with knees bent. Hold arms straight out or overhead, brace core and lean back keeping spine as straight as possible.

_____ Reps _____ Sets _____X Day _____Hold		_____ Reps _____ Sets _____X Day _____Hold
57	Notes:	**58**	Notes:

Starting Position

LEAN BACK WITH TWIST

Start in an upright seated position with knees bent. Hold arms straight out, brace core and lean back keeping spine as straight as possible. Rotate trunk/arms to one side and then repeat to the other side.

Starting Position

LEAN BACK WITH TWIST – BOSU

Start in an upright seated position on Bosu with knees bent. Hold arms straight out, brace core and lean back keeping spine as straight as possible. Rotate trunk/arms to one side - repeat to the other side

_____ Reps _____ Sets _____X Day _____Hold		_____ Reps _____ Sets _____X Day _____Hold
59	Notes:	**60**	Notes:

CRUNCHY FROG

Sit on floor or edge of couch/bench. Lean back and with arms wide apart and legs straight. Next, bring knees towards chest and arms forward and return to starting position.

SEATED BIKE - FORWARD AND BACKWARDS

Sit on floor and lean back. With arms on floor or off ground, peddle feet forward for 15-30 repetitions, rest and then reverse. *Progress by moving hands forward near hips or remove arm support*

Abdominal Crunch Variations

	_____ Reps	_____ Sets	_____ X Day	_____ Hold

61 Notes:

Starting
Position

CRUNCH – ARMS OUT

Lie on your back with your arms outstretched forward, brace core and curl up lifting your shoulder blades off the ground. Exhale as you come up and squeeze/tighten your abdominal muscles.

	_____ Reps	_____ Sets	_____ X Day	_____ Hold

62 Notes:

Starting
Position

CRUNCH – ARMS OUT - BOSU

Lie on your back on Bosu with your arms outstretched forward, brace core and curl up lifting your shoulder blades off the ground. Exhale as you come up and squeeze/tighten your abdominal muscles.

	_____ Reps	_____ Sets	_____ X Day	_____ Hold

63 Notes:

Starting
Position

CRUNCH – ARMS IN BACK OF HEAD

Lie on your back with your arms behind your head, brace core and curl up lifting your shoulder blades off the ground. Exhale as you come up and squeeze/tighten your abdominal muscles. Do not pull on your neck/head.

	_____ Reps	_____ Sets	_____ X Day	_____ Hold

64 Notes:

CRUNCH – ARMS IN BACK OF HEAD - BOSU

Lie on your back on Bosu with your arms behind your head, brace core and curl up lifting your shoulder blades off the ground. Exhale as you come up and squeeze/tighten your abdominal muscles. Do not pull on your neck/head.

_____ Reps _____ Sets _____X Day _____Hold

65 Notes:

OBLIQUE CRUNCH

Lie on your back with one or both hands in back of head. Brace core and curl up targeting elbow to opposite knee as shown. Keep shoulders off floor. Exhale as you come up and squeeze/tighten your abdominal muscles. Do not pull on your neck/head.

_____ Reps _____ Sets _____X Day _____Hold

66 Notes:

OBLIQUE CRUNCH - BOSU

Lie back on Bosu with one or both hands in back of head. Brace core and curl up targeting elbow to opposite knee as shown. Keep shoulders off Bosu. Exhale as you come up and squeeze/tighten your abdominal muscles. Do not pull on your neck/head.

_____ Reps _____ Sets _____X Day _____Hold

67 Notes:

90 DEGREE CRUNCH

Lie on your back with legs straight in air. Reach your hands towards toes, crunching shoulders off ground. Exhale as you come up and squeeze/tighten your abdominal muscles.

_____ Reps _____ Sets _____X Day _____Hold

68 Notes:

BALL CRUNCH – Can put legs on seat of chair

Lie on back with legs up on ball so knees and hips are at ~ 90 degrees. Cross hands over chest or behind head. Brace core and curl up lifting your shoulder blades off the ground. Exhale as you come up and squeeze/tighten your abdominal muscles. Do not pull on your neck/head.

_____ Reps _____ Sets _____X Day _____Hold

69 | Notes:

Starting Position

CURL UPS – ARMS ON LEGS - EXERCISE BALL

While sitting on an exercise ball, roll forward so that your back lies against the ball. Put hands on thighs/legs. Brace core and curl up lifting your shoulder blades off the ball. Exhale as you come up and squeeze/tighten your abdominal muscles.

_____ Reps _____ Sets _____X Day _____Hold

70 | Notes:

CURL UPS- ARMS CROSSED IN FRONT - EXERCISE BALL

While sitting on an exercise ball, roll forward so that your back lies against the ball. Cross hands over your chest. Brace core and curl up lifting your shoulder blades off the ball. Exhale as you come up and squeeze/tighten your abdominal muscles.

_____ Reps _____ Sets _____X Day _____Hold

71 | Notes:

CURL UPS – ARMS BEHIND HEAD - EXERCISE BALL

While sitting on an exercise ball, roll forward so that your back lies against the ball. Place your hands behind your head. Brace core and curl up lifting your shoulder blades off the ball. Exhale as you come up and squeeze/tighten your abdominal muscles. Do not pull on your neck/head.

_____ Reps _____ Sets _____X Day _____Hold

72 | Notes:

Starting Position

SUPINE CRUNCH TOUCH - EXERCISE BALL

Lie on the floor with your knees bend and holding a ball over your head. Bring both your knees and ball towards each other above your chest and touch your knees to the ball. Slowly return both to original positions and repeat.

_____ Reps _____ Sets _____ X Day _____ Hold	_____ Reps _____ Sets _____ X Day _____ Hold

73 Notes:

74 Notes:

LOWER ABDOMINAL CRUNCH – WITH or WITHOUT BALL

Sit on a solid surface with or without a ball/pillow between your knees. Maintaining a straight spine, contract your lower abdominals. Lift both knees up. Hold and control movement back to starting position. Repeat. Can be done holding onto surface for added stability with or without ball (3rd picture)

HIGH MARCH CRUNCH

Lift knee towards chest keeping hips forward in a high march position. Continue to alternate sides while standing in place. Exhale as you come up and squeeze/tighten your abdominal muscles.

_____ Reps _____ Sets _____ X Day _____ Hold	_____ Reps _____ Sets _____ X Day _____ Hold

75 Notes:

76 Notes:

Starting

Position

STANDING SIDE CRUNCH

Standing with hip rotated out bring knee up towards same side elbow squeezing your obliques. Continue alternating sides while standing in place. Exhale as you come up and squeeze/tighten muscles.

Starting

Position

STANDING BIKE CRUNCH

Lift knee to chest and rotate pulling opposite elbow towards knee. Continue to alternate sides while standing in place. Exhale as you come up and squeeze/tighten muscles.

Strengthening

Anaerobic - without oxygen: Single repetition with maximum resistance

Lifting lighter weights with a high number of repetitions will result in 'toning', whereas lifting heavier weights with a lower number of repetitions will result in 'bulking up'.

Benefits of strengthening	• Increases muscle fiber size and contractile strength • Increases tendon and ligament strength • Increases bone strength / bone mineral density • Improves hormonal balances-decreased cortisol • Increases Peripheral (PNS) and Central (CNS) Nervous System communication/proprioception • Improves function for ADL's (Activities of Daily Living)
Range of Motion (ROM)	Refers to the distance and direction a joint can move between the flexed position and the extended position (stretching from flexion to extension for physiological gain). It is important to be able to complete full ROM before adding resistance. ***Before strengthening (adding resistance), make sure you can go through full ROM*** unless being followed by an MD or physical/occupational therapist or other professional.
Forms of strengthening exercise	• **Isometric** – Muscles contract with no motion at the joint or change in length of the muscle. The exercises usually consist of maximal effort against an object that does not move, like a wall. • **Isotonic** – Muscles contract with motion at the joint; muscles either lengthen or shorten (*see **concentric/eccentric** below*). Tension is not constant through the range of motion. (During a bicep curl, holding a 5 lb weight, the contraction is not constant during the entire movement). Most common form of isotonic exercises use free weights with either dumbbells or a barbell. • **Concentric** – Muscle shortens, positive phase of lift. Bending the elbow in a bicep curl • **Eccentric** – Muscle lengthens, negative phase of lift or lowering. Straightening the elbow in a bicep curl. • **Isokinetic** – Muscles contract with motion at the joint; muscles either lengthen or shorten. Machines or equipment control the speed of the movement, so tension is constant providing the maximum amount of resistance throughout the entire movement.
Repetition (Reps)	Single cycle of lifting and lowering a weight in a controlled manner, moving through the form of the exercise. Example: 12 Bicep curls per set.
Set	Several repetitions performed one after another with no break between. There can be a number of reps per set and sets per exercise depending on the goal of the individual. Example: 12 reps x3 sets
Rep Maximum (RM)	The number of repetitions one can perform at a certain weight is called the Rep Maximum (RM). For example, if one could perform 10 repetitions with a 75 lbs dumbbell, then their RM for that weight would be 10RM. 1RM is the maximum weight that someone can lift in a given exercise - i.e. a weight that they can only lift once. (*Wikipedia*) (*See Bulk Up or Tone Up Below*)
Bulk up or Tone up	Do you want to 'bulk up' or 'tone up'? Although much of this depends on genetics and your ratio of slow and fast twitch fibers, discussed in the *Endurance* section, it is good to know what your goals are before starting. The average person should be able to perform at about 75% of their maximum resistance for 10 repetitions. If you can do ONE bicep curl with a 20-pound dumbbell/weight, then you should be able to do 10 with a 15 lbs. weight. (See *Set*) 20 lbs. x 75% = 15 lbs. Once you get into a routine, it will be easy for you to know when to increase the weight.

General rule of thumb	<ul><li>Work from the Ground up</li><li>Order: Isometric > ROM > Eccentric > Concentric</li><li>Use assistance before resistance – Start without weight to complete range of motion and then add weight with proper form. *(See ROM above)*</li><li>Add weight: 8-12 reps x 2-3 sets of each exercise at 75% of one repetition maximum (one-rep max).</li><li>Once you reach 12 easily, you can then recheck your one-rep max. If it has increased, then increase your weight as above.</li><li>If you are looking to 'bulk up', perform low repetitions at a higher weight – up to 85-90% of the one-rep maximum. 5-8 reps x 2-3 sets. With increased weight, there is a higher risk of injury.</li><li>If you are looking to 'tone up', perform high repetitions with 65-75% of the one-rep max. 12-20 reps x 2-3 sets.</li><li>Do NOT exercise the same muscle group every day. The muscles need about 48-72 hours to repair. This includes the abdomen. **Muscle strengthening, if you are lifting weights, alternate upper and lower body with isolated abdomen exercises every other day as well. For those working out several days a week, find a schedule that works for you, but give each muscle group 48-72 hours to recover.</li><li>Cardiac/aerobic conditioning can be done daily.</li><li>Breathe!! Always exhale on the exertion. For example, when you are doing a crunch, exhale as you flexing the abs or 'curling'. Do not hold your breath.</li><li>Engage your core. Don't forget what you learned under core and balance.</li></ul>

Duration, Frequency, Intensity and Movement Patterns

Intensity: How *much* mental and physical *effort* it takes to sustain an activity.	This can be done using the target heart rate range THR (optimum exercise intensity levels through beats per minute, talk test or rate of perceived exertion.
Duration: How *long* the training lasts.	The higher the intensity, the shorter the duration. The American College of Sports Medicine guidelines recommend all healthy adults aged 18–65 yr should participate in moderate intensity aerobic physical activity for a minimum of 30 min on five days per week, or vigorous intensity aerobic activity for a minimum of 20 min on three days per week.
Frequency: How *often* the training occurs.	Strength training should be performed every other day or 2-3 days a week. It is important to give each muscle group 48-72 hours to recover. Alternate upper and lower body with isolated abdomen/core exercises every other day. For those working out several days a week, find a schedule that works for you as long as you give each muscle group 48 hours of recovery time.
Movement Patterns and Examples Basic movements that help to increase overall body strengthening	<ul><li>Bend and Lift: Squats, Dead Lifts and Leg presses<ul><li>Picking up item off floor</li></ul></li><li>Single Leg: Step ups, Single leg stance, Lunges<ul><li>Walking up steps</li></ul></li><li>Push: Shoulder press, Bench press, Push up<ul><li>Pushing Shopping cart or Lawn mower</li></ul></li><li>Pull: Lat pull downs, Seated rows<ul><li>Vacuuming, Raking</li></ul></li><li>Rotational<ul><li>Shoveling snow</li></ul></li></ul>

EXERCISE Lower Extremity - Lying & Seated Strengthening and Range of Motion	EXERCISE NUMBER	NOTES
INVERSION – SEATED - ELASTIC BAND	1	
INVERSION – SEATED - ELASTIC BAND - 2	2	
EVERSION – SEATED - ELASTIC BAND	3	
EVERSION – SEATED - ELASTIC BAND - 2	4	
ANKLE PUMPS - SEATED	5	
ANKLE PUMPS – SUPINE or FEET UP ON STOOL	6	
DORSIFLEXION – SEATED - ELASTIC BAND	7	
DORSIFLEXION – SEATED - ELASTIC BAND - 2	8	
PLANTARFLEXION - STRAP	9	
PLANTARFLEXION - SEATED – ELASTIC BAND	10	
HEEL SLIDES - SUPINE	11	
HEEL SLIDES - RESISTED EXTENSION – ELASTIC BAND	12	
QUAD SET –ISOMETRIC	13	
QUAD SET WITH TOWEL UNDER HEEL - ISOMETRIC	14	
SHORT ARC QUAD (SAQ) – SELF ASSISTED	15	
SHORT ARC QUAD - (SAQ)	16	
KNEE EXTENSION - SELF ASSISTED	17	
PARTIAL ARC QUAD - LOW SEAT	18	
LONG ARC QUAD (LAQ) – LOW SEAT (90 deg)	19	
LONG ARC QUAD (LAQ) – LOW SEAT - ANKLE WEIGHTS	20	
LONG ARC QUAD (LAQ) - HIGH SEAT	21	
LONG ARC QUAD (LAQ) - HIGH SEAT - ANKLE WEIGHTS	22	
LONG ARC QUAD - ELASTIC BAND – HAND HELD	23	
LONG ARC QUAD - ELASTIC BAND	24	

EXERCISE Lower Extremity - Lying & Seated Strengthening and Range of Motion	EXERCISE NUMBER	NOTES
HAMSTRING CURLS - PRONE - ASSISTED	25	
HAMSTRING CURLS - PRONE	26	
HAMSTRING CURLS - - PRONE - WEIGHTS	27	
HAMSTRING CURLS – PRONE - ELASTIC BAND	28	
HAMSTRING CURLS – ELASTIC BAND	29	
HAMSTRING CURLS – ELASTIC BAND - 2	30	
HAMSTRING CURLS ON BALL	31	
HAMSTRING CURLS - SINGLE LEG - EXERCISE BALL	32	
HIP FLEXION ISOMETRIC	33	
HIP FLEXION ISOMETRIC BILATERAL	34	
HIP FLEXION – ISOMETRIC	35	
STRAIGHT LEG RAISE (SLR)	36	
STRAIGHT LEG RAISE (SLR) – ANKLE WEIGHTS	37	
STRAIGHT LEG RAISE (SLR) - ELASTIC BAND	38	
SEATED MARCHING	39	
SEATED MARCHING - ELASTIC BAND	40	
HIP EXTENSION - PRONE	41	
HIP EXTENSION – PRONE – ANKLE WEIGHTS	42	
HIP EXTENSION – PRONE – ELASTIC BAND	43	
HIP EXTENSION – QUADRUPED	44	
HIP ABDUCTION - SUPINE	45	
HIP ABDUCTION - SUPINE – ANKLE WEIGHTS	46	
HIP ABDUCTION – SUPINE - ELASTIC BAND	47	
HIP ABDUCTION / CLAMS– SUPINE - ELASTIC BAND	48	
MODIFIED HIP ABDUCTION – SIDELYING	49	

EXERCISE Lower Extremity - Lying & Seated Strengthening and Range of Motion	EXERCISE NUMBER	NOTES
HIP ABDUCTION – SIDELYING	50	
HIP ABDUCTION – SIDELYING - WEIGHTS	51	
HIP ABDUCTION – SIDELYING - ELASTIC BAND	52	
CLAM SHELLS	53	
SIDELYING CLAM - ELASTIC BAND	54	
HIP ABDUCTION - FIRE HYDRANT - QUADRUPED	55	
HIP ABDUCTION - FIRE HYDRANT – QUADRUPED - ELASTIC BAND	56	
HIP ABDUCTION - SEATED - STRAIGHT LEG	57	
HIP ABDUCTION - SEATED - STRAIGHT LEG – ANKLE WEIGHT	58	
HIP ABDUCTION - SINGLE- SEATED	59	
HIP ABDUCTION - SINGLE- SEATED – ELASTIC BAND	60	
HIP ABDUCTION - BILATERAL- SEATED	61	
HIP ABDUCTION - BILATERAL- SEATED - ELASTIC BAND	62	
HIP ADDUCTION SQUEEZE – SUPINE – KNEES BENT	63	
HIP ADDUCTION SQUEEZE – SUPINE – LEGS STRAIGHT	64	
HIP ADDUCTION - SIDELYING	65	
INTERNAL ROTATION - HEEL SQUEEZE - ISOMETRIC	67	
HIP INTERNAL ROTATION - SUPINE	68	
REVERSE CLAMS - SIDELYING	69	
REVERSE CLAMS - SIDELYING - ELASTIC BAND	70	
HIP INTERNAL ROTATION - SEATED	71	
HIP INTERNAL ROTATION - ELASTIC BAND	72	
HIP EXTERNAL ROTATION - SUPINE	73	

EXERCISE Lower Extremity - Lying & Seated Strengthening and Range of Motion	EXERCISE NUMBER	NOTES
HIP EXTERNAL ROTATION - ELASTIC BAND	74	
HIP ROTATIONS – BILATERAL - SIDELYING	75	
HIP ROTATION - SEATED - BALL and ELASTIC BAND	76	
PRESS – BILATERAL – ELASTIC BAND	77	
PRESS – SINGLE LEG – ELASTIC BAND	78	
HIP HIKE - STANDING	79	
HIP HIKE – KNEELING	80	
GLUTE SETS - PRONE	81	
GLUTE SET - SUPINE	82	
GLUTE SQUEEZE - SITTING	83	
PT (MAX/MEDIUS)	84	

LOWER EXTREMITY - Range Of Motion > Isometric > Strength
Lying and Seated
Inversion (IV) / Eversion (EV)

_____ Reps _____ Sets _____X Day _____Hold	_____ Reps _____ Sets _____X Day _____Hold

1 | Notes:

2 | Notes:

INVERSION – SEATED - ELASTIC BAND

In a seated position, cross your legs and using an elastic band attached to your foot, hook it under your opposite foot and up to your hand. Draw the resisted foot inward. Keep your heel in contact with the floor the entire time.

INVERSION – SEATED - ELASTIC BAND - 2

In a seated position, use an elastic band secured to a steady object and the other end attached to your foot. Draw the resisted foot inward. Keep your heel in contact with the floor the entire time.

_____ Reps _____ Sets _____X Day _____Hold	_____ Reps _____ Sets _____X Day _____Hold

3 | Notes:

4 | Notes:

EVERSION – SEATED - ELASTIC BAND

In a seated position, use an elastic band attached to your foot, hook it under your opposite foot and up to your hand. Draw the resisted foot outward. Keep your heel in contact with the floor the entire time.

EVERSION – SEATED - ELASTIC BAND - 2

In a seated position, use an elastic band secured to a steady object and the other end attached to your foot. Draw the resisted foot outward. Keep your heel in contact with the floor the entire time.

Dorsiflexion (DF) / Plantarflexion (PF)

_____ Reps _____ Sets _____X Day _____Hold	_____ Reps _____ Sets _____X Day _____Hold

5	Notes:	6	Notes:

ANKLE PUMPS - SEATED

In a seated position keeping feet on the floor, first go up on toes (toes pointed towards the ground – PF). Then point toes up keeping heels on the ground (DF). Alternate back and forth in a pumping motion.

ANKLE PUMPS – SUPINE or FEET UP ON STOOL

Lying or with feet up on stool first point the toes forward (PF) and then back up with toes facing the ceiling. Alternate back and forth in a pumping motion.

_____ Reps _____ Sets _____X Day _____Hold	_____ Reps _____ Sets _____X Day _____Hold

7	Notes:	8	Notes:

DORSIFLEXION – SEATED - ELASTIC BAND

In a seated position, use an elastic band attached to your target foot, hook it under your opposite foot and up to your hand. Draw the band upwards with the resisted foot as shown. Keep your heel in contact with the floor the entire time.

DORSIFLEXION – SEATED - ELASTIC BAND - 2

In a seated position, use an elastic band secured to a steady object and the other end attached to your foot. Draw the resisted foot upward. Keep your heel in contact with the floor the entire time.

	_____ Reps _____ Sets _____X Day _____Hold			_____ Reps _____ Sets _____X Day _____Hold
9	Notes:		**10**	Notes:

PLANTARFLEXION - STRAP

In a seated position, attach one loop of the strap to your foot and hold the other end. Move your foot forward and back at the ankle as shown. Keep your heel in contact with the floor the entire time.

PLANTARFLEXION - SEATED – ELASTIC BAND

In a seated position, hold an elastic band and attach the other end to your foot. Press your foot downward towards the floor. Keep your heel in contact with the floor the entire time.

Heel Slides

	_____ Reps _____ Sets _____X Day _____Hold			_____ Reps _____ Sets _____X Day _____Hold
11	Notes:		**12**	Notes:

HEEL SLIDES - SUPINE

Lie on your back with knees straight and slide the target heel towards your buttock as you bend your knee. Hold a gentle stretch in this position and then return to original position.

Starting Position

HEEL SLIDES - RESISTED EXTENSION – ELASTIC BAND

Long sit with band around bottom of target foot. Slide the target heel towards your buttock as you bend your knee. Push your foot to straighten knee against resistance to the original position.

Quadriceps (QUAD) / Knee Extension

_____ Reps _____ Sets _____X Day _____Hold	_____ Reps _____ Sets _____X Day _____Hold
13 Notes:	**14** Notes:

QUAD SET –ISOMETRIC

Tighten your top thigh muscle as you attempt to press the back of your knee downward towards the table. Hold 5-10 seconds. Repeat.

Starting Position

QUAD SET WITH TOWEL UNDER HEEL - ISOMETRIC

Lying or sitting with a small towel roll under your ankle, tighten your top thigh muscle to press the back of your knee downward towards the ground. Hold 5-10 seconds. Repeat.

_____ Reps _____ Sets _____X Day _____Hold	_____ Reps _____ Sets _____X Day _____Hold
15 Notes:	**16** Notes:

Starting Position

SHORT ARC QUAD (SAQ) – SELF ASSISTED

Place a rolled-up towel or other rounded object under your knee. Hook one foot under the other to assist the affected leg. Slowly straighten your knee as your raise up your foot tightening the top thigh muscle.

SHORT ARC QUAD - (SAQ) - Can add ankle weight

Place a rolled-up towel or object under your knee and slowly straighten your knee as your raise up your foot tightening the top thigh muscle. Flex your foot to increase the stretch.

	_____ Reps _____ Sets _____ X Day _____ Hold
17	**Notes:**

KNEE EXTENSION - SELF ASSISTED

In a seated position, place the unaffected leg under the target leg. Use the unaffected leg to assist the target leg up to a straightened knee position.

	_____ Reps _____ Sets _____ X Day _____ Hold
18	**Notes:**

PARTIAL ARC QUAD - LOW SEAT - Can add ankle weight

Sit with your knee in a semi bent position and your heel touching the ground and then slowly straighten your knee as you raise your foot upwards as shown. Lower your foot back down slowly controlling the muscle until your heel touches the ground and then repeat.

	_____ Reps _____ Sets _____ X Day _____ Hold
19	**Notes:**

LONG ARC QUAD (LAQ) – LOW SEAT (90 deg)

Sit with your knee in a bent position and then tighten the quadricep. Slowly straighten your knee as you raise your foot upwards as shown. Lower your foot back down to original bent knee position slowly controlling the muscle and then repeat.

	_____ Reps _____ Sets _____ X Day _____ Hold
20	**Notes:**

LONG ARC QUAD (LAQ) – LOW SEAT - ANKLE WEIGHTS

Attach and ankle weight. Sit with your knee in a bent position and then tighten the quadricep. Slowly straighten your knee as you raise your foot upwards as shown. Lower your foot back down to original bent knee position slowly controlling the muscle - repeat.

_____ Reps	_____ Sets	_____ X Day	_____ Hold

21 | **Notes:**

LONG ARC QUAD (LAQ) - HIGH SEAT

Sit with your knee in a bent position and then tighten the quadricep. Slowly straighten your knee as you raise your foot upwards as shown. Lower your foot back down to original bent knee position slowly controlling the muscle and then repeat.

_____ Reps	_____ Sets	_____ X Day	_____ Hold

22 | **Notes:**

LONG ARC QUAD (LAQ) - HIGH SEAT - ANKLE WEIGHTS

Attach and ankle weight. Sit with your knee in a bent position and then tighten the quadricep. Slowly straighten your knee as you raise your foot upwards as shown. Lower your foot back down to original bent knee position slowly controlling the muscle and then repeat.

_____ Reps	_____ Sets	_____ X Day	_____ Hold

23 | **Notes:**

LONG ARC QUAD - ELASTIC BAND – HANDHELD

Attach a looped elastic band to your ankle and to the opposite foot or hold with your hand. Sit with your knee in a bent position and then tighten the quadricep. Draw your lower leg upwards to a straighten knee position while your other foot or hand secures the band. Lower your foot back down to original bent knee position slowly controlling the muscle and then repeat.

_____ Reps	_____ Sets	_____ X Day	_____ Hold

24 | **Notes:**

LONG ARC QUAD - ELASTIC BAND

Attach a looped elastic band to your ankle and to a steady object behind you. Sit with your knee in a bent position and then tighten the quadricep. Draw your lower leg upwards to a straightened knee position. Lower your foot back down to original bent knee position slowly controlling the muscle and then repeat.

Hamstrings

	_____ Reps _____ Sets _____ X Day _____ Hold
25	**Notes:**

HAMSTRING CURLS - PRONE - ASSISTED

Lie face down and hook one foot under the other to assist the affected leg. Bend the target leg with the assistance of your unaffected leg.

	_____ Reps _____ Sets _____ X Day _____ Hold
26	**Notes:**

HAMSTRING CURLS - PRONE

Lie face down and slowly bend your knee as you bring your foot towards your buttock.

	_____ Reps _____ Sets _____ X Day _____ Hold
27	**Notes:**

HAMSTRING CURLS - - PRONE - WEIGHTS

Attach and ankle weight. Lie face down and slowly bend your knee as you bring your foot towards your buttock.

	_____ Reps _____ Sets _____ X Day _____ Hold
28	**Notes:**

HAMSTRING CURLS – PRONE - ELASTIC BAND

Attach an elastic band around your foot and opposite ankle as shown. While lying face down, slowly bend your target knee as you bring your foot towards your buttock. Keep your other foot on the floor to fixate the band.

	_____ Reps _____ Sets _____X Day _____Hold
29	Notes:

HAMSTRING CURLS – ELASTIC BAND

Sit and use an elastic band secured to a steady object and the other end attached to your ankle. Bend your knee and draw back your foot.

	_____ Reps _____ Sets _____X Day _____Hold
30	Notes:

HAMSTRING CURLS – ELASTIC BAND - 2

Attach a looped elastic band to your ankle and to the opposite foot while one leg is propped on stool or another raised object. Draw your lower leg downwards to a bent knee position while your other ankle anchors the band on the chair.

	_____ Reps _____ Sets _____X Day _____Hold
31	Notes:

HAMSTRING CURLS ON BALL – can add ankle weight.

Lie prone on an exercise ball as shown. Slowly bend your knee as you bring your foot towards your buttock.

	_____ Reps _____ Sets _____X Day _____Hold
32	Notes: **Advanced**

Starting Position

HAMSTRING CURLS - SINGLE LEG - EXERCISE BALL

Lie on the floor and place your heel on an exercise ball.
Lift your buttocks and then bend your knees to draw the ball towards your buttocks. Keep your buttocks elevated off the floor the entire time.

Hip Flexion

	_____ Reps _____ Sets _____X Day _____Hold
33	**Notes:**

HIP FLEXION ISOMETRIC

Lie on your back, lift up your knee and press it into your hand. Hold. Return to the original position and repeat.

HIP FLEXION ISOMETRIC - ALTERNATING
Lie on your back, lift up your knee and press it into your hand. Hold. Return to the original position and repeat on the other side.

	_____ Reps _____ Sets _____X Day _____Hold
34	**Notes:**

HIP FLEXION ISOMETRIC BILATERAL

Lie on your back, lift up your knees and press them into your hands. Hold. Return to the original position and repeat.

	_____ Reps _____ Sets _____X Day _____Hold
35	**Notes:**

HIP FLEXION – ISOMETRIC - Can use towel roll for comfort

While standing in front of a wall, draw your knee forward and press it into the wall. Place a folded towel between your knee and the wall for comfort if needed.

	_____ Reps _____ Sets _____X Day _____Hold
36	**Notes:**

STRAIGHT LEG RAISE (SLR)

Lie on your back, tighten the quad of the target leg and lift up with a straight knee. Keep the opposite knee bent with the foot planted on the ground. (see #37 for starting position)

_____ Reps _____ Sets _____X Day _____Hold

37 | Notes:

Starting

Position

STRAIGHT LEG RAISE (SLR) – ANKLE WEIGHTS

Attach ankle weights. Lie on your back and lift up your leg with a straight knee. Keep the opposite knee bent with the foot planted on the ground

_____ Reps _____ Sets _____X Day _____Hold

38 | Notes:

STRAIGHT LEG RAISE (SLR) - ELASTIC BAND

Lie on your back with an elastic band looped around your ankles, lift the target leg upwards.

_____ Reps _____ Sets _____X Day _____Hold

39 | Notes:

SEATED MARCHING - can add ankle weights for resistance

Sit in a chair and move a knee upward, set it back down and then alternate to the other side

_____ Reps _____ Sets _____X Day _____Hold

40 | Notes:

SEATED MARCHING - ELASTIC BAND

Sit in a chair with an elastic band wrapped around your thighs. Move a knee upward, set it back down and then alternate to the other side.

Hip Extension

	_____ Reps _____ Sets _____ X Day _____ Hold		_____ Reps _____ Sets _____ X Day _____ Hold
41	Notes:	**42**	Notes:

HIP EXTENSION - PRONE

Lie face down with your knee straight and slowly lift up leg off the ground. Maintain a straight knee the entire time.

HIP EXTENSION – PRONE – ANKLE WEIGHTS

Attach ankle weights. Lie face down with your knee straight and slowly lift up leg off the ground. Maintain a straight knee the entire time.

	_____ Reps _____ Sets _____ X Day _____ Hold		_____ Reps _____ Sets _____ X Day _____ Hold
43	Notes:	**44**	Notes:

HIP EXTENSION – PRONE – ELASTIC BAND

Lie on your stomach with an elastic band looped around your ankles and lift the targeted leg upwards. Maintain a straight knee the entire time.

HIP EXTENSION – QUADRUPED with or without ankle weights

Start in a crawl position and then raise your leg up behind you as shown. Keep your knee bent at 90 degrees the entire time.

Hip Abduction (ABD)

	_____ Reps _____ Sets _____X Day _____Hold
45	**Notes:**

HIP ABDUCTION - SUPINE

Lie on your back and slowly bring your leg out to the side. Return to original position and repeat. Keep your knee straight the entire time.

	_____ Reps _____ Sets _____X Day _____Hold
46	**Notes:**

HIP ABDUCTION - SUPINE – ANKLE WEIGHTS

Attach and weights. Lie on your back and slowly bring your leg up slightly and then out to the side. Return to original position and repeat. Keep your knee straight the entire time.

	_____ Reps _____ Sets _____X Day _____Hold
47	**Notes:**

HIP ABDUCTION – SUPINE - ELASTIC BAND

Lie on your back and slowly bring your leg out to the side. Return to original position and repeat. Keep your knee straight the entire time.

	_____ Reps _____ Sets _____X Day _____Hold
48	**Notes:**

HIP ABDUCTION / CLAMS– SUPINE - ELASTIC BAND

Lie down on your back with your knees bent. Place an elastic band around your knees and then draw your knees apart. Return to original position and repeat.

	_____ Reps _____ Sets _____X Day _____Hold
49	**Notes:**

MODIFIED HIP ABDUCTION – SIDELYING can add weights

Lie on your side and slowly lift up your top leg to the side. The bottom leg can be bent to stabilize your body. Keep your knee straight and maintain your toes pointed forward the entire time. Keep your leg in-line with your body. Return to original position and repeat.

	_____ Reps _____ Sets _____X Day _____Hold
50	**Notes:**

HIP ABDUCTION – SIDELYING

Lie on your side and slowly lift up your top leg to the side. Keep your knee straight and maintain your toes pointed forward the entire time. Keep your leg in-line with your body. Return to original position and repeat.

	_____ Reps _____ Sets _____X Day _____Hold
51	**Notes:**

HIP ABDUCTION – SIDELYING - WEIGHTS

Attach ankle weights. Lie on your side and slowly lift up your top leg to the side. Keep your knee straight and maintain your toes pointed forward the entire time. Keep your leg in-line with your body. Return to original position and repeat.

	_____ Reps _____ Sets _____X Day _____Hold
52	**Notes:**

HIP ABDUCTION – SIDELYING - ELASTIC BAND

Lie on your side with an elastic band looped around your ankles. Lift the top leg upwards keeping your knee straight and maintaining your toes pointed forward the entire time. Keep your leg in-line with your body. Return to original position and repeat.

_____ Reps _____ Sets _____X Day _____Hold

53	Notes:

Starting Position

CLAM SHELLS

Lie on your side with your knees bent, draw up the top knee while keeping contact of your feet together. Do not let your pelvis roll back during the lifting movement.

_____ Reps _____ Sets _____X Day _____Hold

54	Notes:

Starting Position

SIDELYING CLAM - ELASTIC BAND

Lie on your side with your knees bent and an elastic band wrapped around your knees, draw up the top knee while keeping contact of your feet together as shown. Do not let your pelvis roll back during the lifting movement.

_____ Reps _____ Sets _____X Day _____Hold

55	Notes:

Starting Position

HIP ABDUCTION - FIRE HYDRANT - QUADRUPED

Start in a crawl position and raise your leg out to the side as shown. Maintain a straight upper and mid back.

_____ Reps _____ Sets _____X Day _____Hold

56	Notes:

Starting Position

HIP ABDUCTION - FIRE HYDRANT – QUADRUPED - ELASTIC BAND

Start in a crawl position with an elastic band around your thighs. Raise your leg out to the side as shown. Maintain a straight upper and mid back.

	_____ Reps _____ Sets _____ X Day _____ Hold
57	Notes:

HIP ABDUCTION - SEATED - STRAIGHT LEG

Sit close to the edge of a chair with your target leg straight at the knee. Move your target leg to the side lifting slightly off the ground and then return to straight ahead.. You can slide your heel across the floor as you move and then return to straight ahead if unable to lift. Maintain your toes pointed up the entire time.

	_____ Reps _____ Sets _____ X Day _____ Hold
58	Notes:

HIP ABDUCTION - SEATED - STRAIGHT LEG – ANKLE WEIGHT

Attach an ankle weight. Sit close to the edge of a chair with your target leg straight at the knee. Move your target leg to the side lifting slightly off the ground and then return to straight ahead. Maintain your toes pointed up the entire time.

	_____ Reps _____ Sets _____ X Day _____ Hold
59	Notes:

HIP ABDUCTION - SINGLE- SEATED

Sit close to the edge of a chair with knees bent and both feet on the floor. Move your target knee out to the side as shown and then return to straight ahead. Maintain contact of your feet on the floor the entire time.

	_____ Reps _____ Sets _____ X Day _____ Hold
60	Notes:

HIP ABDUCTION - SINGLE- SEATED – ELASTIC BAND

With band tied around the thighs, sit close to the edge of a chair with knees bent and both feet on the floor. Move your target knee out to the side as shown and then return to straight ahead. Maintain contact of your feet on the floor the entire time.tact of your feet on the floor the entire time.

	_____ Reps _____ Sets _____X Day _____Hold		_____ Reps _____ Sets _____X Day _____Hold
61	Notes:	62	Notes:

HIP ABDUCTION - BILATERAL- SEATED

Sit close to the edge of a chair with knees bent and both feet on the floor. Move your knees out to the side as shown and then return to straight ahead. Maintain contact of your feet on the floor the entire time.

HIP ABDUCTION - BILATERAL- SEATED - ELASTIC BAND

Sit close to the edge of a chair with an elastic band wrapped around your knees. Move both knees to the sides to separate your legs. Keep contact of your feet on the floor the entire time.

Hip Adduction (ADD)

	_____ Reps _____ Sets _____X Day _____Hold		_____ Reps _____ Sets _____X Day _____Hold
63	Notes:	64	Notes:

HIP ADDUCTION SQUEEZE – SUPINE – KNEES BENT

Lie on your back with legs bent and place a rolled up towel, ball or pillow between your knees. Press your knees together so that you squeeze the object firmly. Hold, release and repeat.

HIP ADDUCTION SQUEEZE – SUPINE – LEGS STRAIGHT

Lie on your back and place a rolled up towel, ball or pillow between your knees. Squeeze the object with your knees. Hold, release and repeat.

	_____ Reps _____ Sets _____X Day _____Hold		_____ Reps _____ Sets _____X Day _____Hold
65	Notes:	66	Notes:

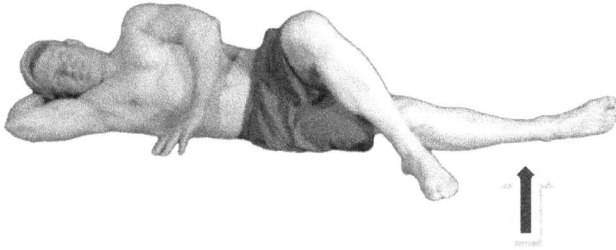

HIP ADDUCTION - SIDELYING

Lie on your side, slowly lift up your bottom leg towards the ceiling. Keep your knee straight the entire time. Your top leg should be bent at the knee and your foot planted on the ground supporting your body.

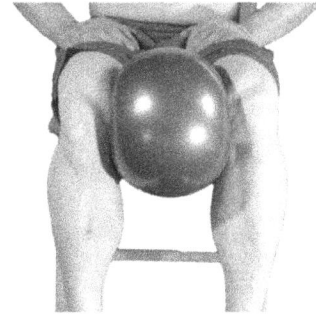

BALL SQUEEZE - SEATED

Sit and place a rolled-up towel, ball or pillow between your knees and squeeze the object firmly. Hold, release and repeat.

Hip Internal Rotation (IR)

	_____ Reps _____ Sets _____X Day _____Hold		_____ Reps _____ Sets _____X Day _____Hold
67	Notes:	68	Notes:

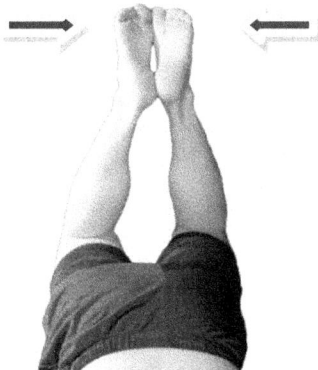

INTERNAL ROTATION - HEEL SQUEEZE - ISOMETRIC

Lie face down, spead your knees apart and press your heels together. Hold, release and repeat.

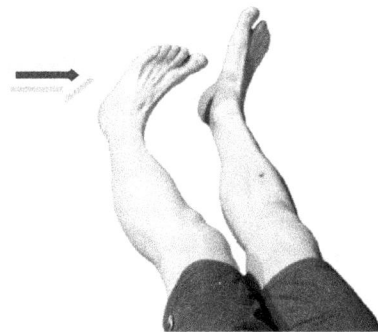

HIP INTERNAL ROTATION - SUPINE

Lie on your back with your knees straight, roll your hip in so that your toes point inward. Be sure that your knee cap faces inward as well.

_____ Reps _____ Sets _____ X Day _____ Hold

69 Notes:

Starting Position

REVERSE CLAMS - SIDELYING

Lie on your side with your knees bent and raise your top foot towards the ceiling while keeping contact of your knees together. Lower back down to original position. Do not let your pelvis roll forward during the lifting movement.

_____ Reps _____ Sets _____ X Day _____ Hold

70 Notes:

Starting Position

REVERSE CLAMS - SIDELYING - ELASTIC BAND

Lie on your side with your knees bent and an elastic band around your ankles. Raise your top foot towards the ceiling while keeping contact of your knees together. Lower back down to original position. Do not let your pelvis roll forward during the lifting movement.

_____ Reps _____ Sets _____ X Day _____ Hold

71 Notes:

HIP INTERNAL ROTATION - SEATED

Sit on a chair with your legs spread apart and feet planted on the ground. Use your hand on the inside of your knee to resist the movement inward.

_____ Reps _____ Sets _____ X Day _____ Hold

72 Notes:

HIP INTERNAL ROTATION - ELASTIC BAND - High chair

Attach one end of an elastic band at your ankle and the other to a sturdy object. Pull away from your other leg while keeping your thigh from moving.

Hip External Rotation (ER)

	_____ Reps _____ Sets _____ X Day _____ Hold		_____ Reps _____ Sets _____ X Day _____ Hold
73	Notes:	**74**	Notes:

HIP EXTERNAL ROTATION - SUPINE

Lie on your back with your knees straight and roll your hip out so that your toes point outward. Be sure that your knee cap faces outward as well.

HIP EXTERNAL ROTATION - ELASTIC BAND

Sit and use an elastic band secured to a steady object and the other end attached to your ankle from the side.
Pull towards your other leg while keeping your thigh from moving across the table.

Bilateral Hip Rotation

	_____ Reps _____ Sets _____ X Day _____ Hold		_____ Reps _____ Sets _____ X Day _____ Hold
75	Notes:	**76**	Notes:

HIP ROTATIONS – BILATERAL - SIDELYING

Lie on your side in fetal position with knees and hips bent.
Slowly raise up both lower legs and feet as shown.
Your feet and knees should be touching the entire time.

HIP ROTATION - SEATED - BALL and ELASTIC BAND – High chair

Sit and place a rolled-up towel, ball or pillow between your knees and an elastic band around your ankles. Squeeze the ball, sustain and hold. Next, pull the band as you move your feet apart from each other.

Leg Press

	_____ Reps _____ Sets _____ X Day _____ Hold			_____ Reps _____ Sets _____ X Day _____ Hold
77	Notes:		78	Notes:

Starting Position

PRESS – BILATERAL – ELASTIC BAND

Lie on back put elastic band on bottom of both feet. Start with knees bent and push with feet to straighten both legs.

PRESS – SINGLE LEG – ELASTIC BAND

Lie on back put elastic band on bottom of one foot. Start with knees bent and push with foot to straighten leg.

Hip Hikes (Gluteus Medius)

	_____ Reps _____ Sets _____ X Day _____ Hold			_____ Reps _____ Sets _____ X Day _____ Hold
79	Notes:		80	Notes:

HIP HIKE - STANDING on Step or Pad

Stand with one foot on a step or pad and the other hanging off as shown. Raise and lower the side of your pelvis that is hanging off the edge.

HIP HIKE – KNEELING on towel or pad

Kneel on both knees with one knee on a folded towel or pad. Raise and lower the side of your pelvis that is not on the towel/pad.

Glutes (Glute Max)

_____ Reps _____ Sets _____ X Day _____ Hold	_____ Reps _____ Sets _____ X Day _____ Hold
81 Notes:	**82** Notes:

GLUTE SETS - PRONE

Lie face down, squeeze your buttocks and hold. Repeat.

GLUTE SET - SUPINE

Lie on your back, squeeze your buttocks and hold. Repeat.

_____ Reps _____ Sets _____ X Day _____ Hold	_____ Reps _____ Sets _____ X Day _____ Hold
83 Notes:	**84** Notes:

GLUTE SQUEEZE - SITTING

While sitting, squeeze your buttocks and hold. Repeat.

GLUTE SCULPT (MAX/MEDIUS)

Lie on your side leaning towards your stomach. Bend leg on target side, raise up and hold.

EXERCISE Upper Extremity Strengthening and Range of Motion	EXERCISE NUMBER	NOTES
ELBOW FLEXION EXTENSION - SUPINE	1	
ELBOW FLEXION / EXTENSION - GRAVITY ELIMINATED	2	
BICEPS CURLS – ALTERNATING	3	
BICEPS CURL - SELF FIXATION – ELASTIC BAND	4	
SEATED BICEPS CURLS - ALTERNATING	5	
SEATED BICEPS CURLS - BILATERAL	6	
CONCENTRATION CURLS – SITTING	7	
PREACHER CURL ON BALL	8	
BICEPS CURLS	9	
BICEPS CURLS - RADIOBRACHIALIS - HAMMER CURL	10	
BICEPS CURLS - BRACHIALIS	11	
BICEPS CURLS – ROTATE OUTWARD	12	
BICEPS CURLS – ONE ARM - ELASTIC BAND	13	
BICEPS CURLS – BILATERAL - ELASTIC BAND	14	
BICEPS CURLS - RADIOBRACHIALIS - HAMMER CURL – ONE ARM - ELASTIC BAND	15	
BICEPS CURLS - RADIOBRACHIALIS - HAMMER CURL – BILATERAL - ELASTIC BAND	16	
BICEPS CURLS – BRACHIALIS - ONE ARM - ELASTIC BAND	17	
BICEPS CURL – BRACHIALIS – BILATERAL - ELASTIC BAND	18	
TRICEPS - SELF FIXATION - ELASTIC BAND	19	
OVERHEAD TRICEPS - SELF FIXATION –SEATED OR STANDING - ELASTIC BAND	20	
TRICEP EXTENSION – SITTING OR STANDING - WEIGHT	21	
TRICEP EXTENSION – SITTING OR STANDING – BILATERAL - WEIGHT	22	
ELBOW EXTENSION - BALL	23	

EXERCISE Upper Extremity Strengthening and Range of Motion	EXERCISE NUMBER	NOTES
ELBOW EXTENSION - SKULL CRUSHER - BALL	24	
TRICEPS - ELASTIC BAND	25	
TRICEPS - BENT OVER	26	
CHAIR DIPS / PUSH UPS	27	
DIPS OFF CHAIR	28	
PENDULUM SHOULDER FORWARD/BACK	29	
PENDULUM SHOULDER – SIDE TO SIDE	30	
PENDULUM SHOULDER CIRCLES	31	
PENDULUMS - SUPINE	32	
ISOMETRIC FLEXION	33	
SHOULDER FLEXION – SIDELYING	34	
FLEXION – SUPINE - SINGLE OR BILATERAL	35	
FLEXION – SUPINE – SINGLE OR BILATERAL - WEIGHT	36	
FLEXION – SUPINE - DOWEL	37	
FLEXION – SUPINE - DOWEL - Weight	38	
FLEXION - SELF FIXATION – ELASTIC BAND	39	
FLEXION – ELASTIC BAND	40	
FLEXION - STANDING - PALMS DOWN / OVERHAND DOWEL	41	
FLEXION - STANDING - PALMS UP / UNDERHAND DOWEL	42	
FLEXION – PALMS FACING INWARD	43	
FLEXION – PALMS DOWN	44	
V RAISE	45	
V RAISE – WEIGHTS	46	
MILITARY PRESS – DOWEL	47	
MILITARY PRESS - FREE WEIGHTS	48	

EXERCISE Upper Extremity Strengthening and Range of Motion	EXERCISE NUMBER	NOTES
ISOMETRIC EXTENSION	49	
PRONE EXTENSION - EXERCISE BALL	50	
SHOULDER EXTENSION - STANDING	51	
SHOULDER EXTENSION - STANDING - WEIGHTS	52	
EXTENSION – STANDING – DOWEL	53	
EXTENSION - SELF FIXATION - ELASTIC BAND	54	
EXTENSION - ELASTIC BAND	55	
EXTENSION - BILATERAL - ELASTIC BAND	56	
INTERNAL ROTATION – ISOMETRIC	57	
INTERNAL ROTATION - ISOMETRIC- ELEVATED	58	
INTERNAL ROTATION - SIDELYING	59	
INTERNAL ROTATION - ELASTIC BAND	60	
INTERNAL / EXTERNAL ROTATION - STANDING – DOWEL	61	
INTERNAL ROTATION – DOWEL	62	
EXTERNAL ROTATION - ISOMETRIC	63	
EXTERNAL ROTATION - ISOMETRIC – ELEVATED	64	
EXTERNAL ROTATION WITH TOWEL - SIDELYING	65	
EXTERNAL ROTATION – 90/90 - WEIGHTS	66	
EXTERNAL ROTATION - BILATERAL - ELASTIC BAND	67	
EXTERNAL ROTATION - ELASTIC BAND	68	
ADDUCTION – ISOMETRIC	69	
ADDUCTION - ELASTIC BAND	70	
ABDUCTION – ISOMETRIC	71	
HORIZONTAL ABDUCTION - DOWEL	72	

EXERCISE Upper Extremity Strengthening and Range of Motion	EXERCISE NUMBER	NOTES
HORIZONTAL ABDUCTION/ADDUCTTION - SUPINE	73	
HORIZONTAL ABDUCTION/ADDUCTTION - SUPINE -WEIGHT	74	
ABDUCTION - SIDELYING	75	
HORIZONTAL ABDUCTION - SIDELYING	76	
ABDUCTION – WEIGHT	77	
ABDUCTION – ELASTIC BAND	78	
HORIZONTAL ABDUCTION – BILATERAL - ELASTIC BAND	79	
90/90 ABDUCTION - WEIGHT	80	
LATERAL RAISES	81	
LATERAL RAISES – LEAN FORWARD	82	
LATERAL RAISES – LEAN FORWARD - ARM ROTATION	83	
FRONTAL RAISE – WEIGHTS	84	
UPRIGHT ROW – WEIGHTS	85	
UPRIGHT ROW – ELASTIC BAND	86	
SHRUGS	87	
SHRUGS - WEIGHTS	88	
SHOULDER ROLLS	89	
SHOULDER ROLLS - WEIGHTS	90	
SCAPULAR RETRACTIONS - BILATERAL	91	
SCAPULAR RETRACTION – SINGLE ARM	92	
ELASTIC BAND SCAPULAR RETRACTIONS WITH MINI SHOULDER EXTENSIONS	93	
PRONE RETRACTION	94	
SCAPULAR PROTRACTION - SUPINE - BILATERAL	95	
SCAPULAR PROTRACTION - SUPINE - WEIGHT	96	

EXERCISE Upper Extremity Strengthening and Range of Motion	EXERCISE NUMBER	NOTES
SCAPULAR PROTRACTION - SUPINE - ELASTIC BAND	97	
SCAPULAR PROTRACTION / TABLE PLANK	98	
CHEST PRESS – SEATED or STANDING - ELASTIC BAND	99	
CHEST PRESS – BALL, FLOOR or BENCH- WEIGHTS	100	
DOWEL PRESS – STANDING	101	
CHEST PRESS – STANDING or SEATED	102	
BENT OVER ROWS	103	
ROWS – PRONE	104	
ROWS - ELASTIC BAND	105	
WIDE ROWS - ELASTIC BAND	106	
LOW ROW – ELASTIC BAND	107	
HIGH ROW – ELASTIC BAND	108	
FLY'S – FLOOR - WEIGHT	109	
FLY'S – BALL or BENCH – WEIGHT	110	
WALL PUSH UPS	111	
WALL PUSH UP - BALL	112	
WALL PUSH UP - Triceps uneven	113	
WALL PUSH UP - Hands inverted	114	
WALL PUSH UP - Narrow	115	
WALL PUSH UP – Wide	116	
PUSH UPS - BALL	117	
PUSH UP - MODIFIED	118	
PUSH UP	119	
PUSH UP -DIAMOND	120	
PUSH UP – MODIFIED - BOSU - UNSTABLE	121	

EXERCISE **Upper Extremity Strengthening and Range of Motion**	EXERCISE NUMBER	NOTES
PUSH UP – BOSU - UNSTABLE	122	
PUSH UP – MODIFIED – INVERTED BOSU - UNSTABLE	123	
PUSH UP – INVERTED BOSU - UNSTABLE	124	

UPPER EXTREMITY - Range Of Motion > Isometric > Strength

Elbow Flexion/Extension

	_____ Reps _____ Sets _____X Day _____Hold		_____ Reps _____ Sets _____X Day _____Hold
1	Notes:	**2**	Notes:

Extension

Flexion

ELBOW FLEXION EXTENSION - SUPINE

Lie on your back and rest your elbow on a small rolled up towel. Bend at your elbow and then lower back down.

Flexion

Extension

ELBOW FLEXION / EXTENSION - GRAVITY ELIMINATED

Sit and hold your arm up with the help of your other arm. Bend and straighten your elbow.

Elbow Flexion (Biceps)

	_____ Reps _____ Sets _____X Day _____Hold		_____ Reps _____ Sets _____X Day _____Hold
3	Notes:	**4**	Notes:

BICEPS CURLS – ALTERNATING

Bend your elbow and move your forearm upwards. As you lower back down, begin bending the opposite elbow upwards.

BICEPS CURL - SELF FIXATION – ELASTIC BAND

Sit and hold an elastic band with one hand. Hold the other end of elastic band with the opposite hand and fixate hand on your knee. Slowly draw up your hand by bending at the elbow. Return to starting position and repeat.

*Can increase resistance by doubling band as shown.

	_____ Reps _____ Sets _____ X Day _____ Hold
5	**Notes:** *Neuropathy/Hands – Precaution holding weights

SEATED BICEPS CURLS - ALTERNATING

Sit in a chair and hold free weights on each thigh. Lift one side while bending at the elbow and squeezing bicep muscle. Perform on one side and then alternate to the other side.

	_____ Reps _____ Sets _____ X Day _____ Hold
6	**Notes:** *Neuropathy/Hands – Precaution holding weights

SEATED BICEPS CURLS - BILATERAL

Sit in a chair and hold free weights on each thigh. Lift both sides while bending at the elbows and squeezing bicep muscles. Lower back down and repeat.

	_____ Reps _____ Sets _____ X Day _____ Hold
7	**Notes:** *Neuropathy/Hands – Precaution holding weights

CONCENTRATION CURLS – SITTING

Sit in a chair, lean slightly forward and hold a free weight with arm straight with elbow on inside of thigh. Bend elbow squeezing bicep muscle. Lower back down - repeat.

	_____ Reps _____ Sets _____ X Day _____ Hold
8	**Notes:** *Neuropathy/Hands – Precaution holding weights

Starting Position

PREACHER CURL ON BALL

Lie on stomach over ball in crawling position. Hold weights in both hands with back of arms against ball. Lift both sides while bending at the elbows and squeezing bicep muscles. Lower back down - repeat.

	_____ Reps _____ Sets _____ X Day _____ Hold		_____ Reps _____ Sets _____ X Day _____ Hold	
9	**Notes:** *Neuropathy/Hands – Precaution holding weights	**10**	**Notes:** *Neuropathy/Hands – Precaution holding weights	

BICEPS CURLS

Holding weights and keeping your arm at your side, draw up your hand by bending at the elbow squeezing bicep muscle. Keep your palm face up the entire time. Can perform set on one side and then other or alternate arms.

BICEPS CURLS - RADIOBRACHIALIS - HAMMER CURL

Holding weights and keeping your arm at your side, draw up your hand by bending at the elbow squeezing bicep muscle. Keep your wrist in a neutral position as shown above the entire time. Can perform set on one side and then other or alternate arms.

	_____ Reps _____ Sets _____ X Day _____ Hold		_____ Reps _____ Sets _____ X Day _____ Hold	
11	**Notes:** *Neuropathy/Hands – Precaution holding weights	**12**	**Notes:** *Neuropathy/Hands – Precaution holding weights	

BICEPS CURLS - BRACHIALIS

Holding weights and keeping your arm at your side, draw up your hand by bending at the elbow squeezing bicep muscle. Keep your palm face down the entire time. Can perform set on one side and then other or alternate arms.

BICEPS CURLS – ROTATE OUTWARD

Holding weights and keeping your arm at your side, draw up your hand by bending at the elbow squeezing bicep muscle. Keep your palm face up the entire time. You can do this one arm at a time or bilateral.

13	_____ Reps _____ Sets _____X Day _____Hold
	Notes:

BICEPS CURLS – ONE ARM - ELASTIC BAND

In a standing position, step on the band with one leg. Keep your arm at your side holding an elastic band and draw up your hand by bending at the elbow squeezing bicep muscle. Keep your palm face up the entire time.

14	_____ Reps _____ Sets _____X Day _____Hold
	Notes:

BICEPS CURLS – BILATERAL - ELASTIC BAND

In a standing position, step on the band with both feet, shoulder width apart. Keep your arms at your side holding an elastic band and draw up your hands by bending at the elbows squeezing bicep muscles. Keep your palms facing upward the entire time.

15	_____ Reps _____ Sets _____X Day _____Hold
	Notes:

BICEPS CURLS - RADIOBRACHIALIS - HAMMER CURL – ONE ARM - ELASTIC BAND

In a standing position, step on the band with one leg. Keep your arm at your side holding an elastic band and draw up your hand by bending at the elbow squeezing bicep muscle. Keep your palm facing inward the entire time.

16	_____ Reps _____ Sets _____X Day _____Hold
	Notes:

BICEPS CURLS - RADIOBRACHIALIS - HAMMER CURL – BILATERAL - ELASTIC BAND

In a standing position, step on the band with both feet, shoulder width apart. Keep your arms at your side holding an elastic band and draw up your hands by bending at the elbows squeezing bicep muscles. Keep your palms facing inward the entire time.

	_____ Reps _____ Sets _____ X Day _____ Hold		_____ Reps _____ Sets _____ X Day _____ Hold
17	Notes:	**18**	Notes:

BICEPS CURLS – BRACHIALIS - ONE ARM - ELASTIC BAND

In a standing position, step on the band with one leg. Keep your arm at your side holding an elastic band and draw up your hand by bending at the elbow squeezing bicep muscle. Keep your palm face down the entire time.

BICEPS CURL – BRACHIALIS – BILATERAL - ELASTIC BAND

In a standing position, step on the band with both feet, shoulder width apart. Keep your arms at your side holding an elastic band and draw up your hands by bending at the elbows squeezing bicep muscles. Keep your palms facing downward the entire time.

Elbow Extension (Triceps)

	_____ Reps _____ Sets _____ X Day _____ Hold		_____ Reps _____ Sets _____ X Day _____ Hold
19	Notes:	**20**	Notes:

TRICEPS - SELF FIXATION - ELASTIC BAND

Hold an elastic band across your chest with the unaffected arm. Pull the band downward with the other arm so that the elbow goes from a bent position to a straightened position as shown.

OVERHEAD TRICEPS - SELF FIXATION –SEATED OR STANDING - ELASTIC BAND

Hold an elastic band with one arm fixated behind back as shown and other hand behind head. Extend elbow with arm overhead and return to starting position.

	_____ Reps _____ Sets _____ X Day _____ Hold
21	**Notes:** *Neuropathy/Hands – Precaution holding weights

Starting

Position

TRICEP EXTENSION – SITTING OR STANDING - WEIGHT

Start with hand behind head holding free weight. Extend your elbow as shown. Maintain your upper arm in an upward direction and only bend and straighten at your elbow.
*Can hold the triceps area with opposite arm to stabilize.

	_____ Reps _____ Sets _____ X Day _____ Hold
22	**Notes:** *Neuropathy/Hands – Precaution holding weights

Starting

Position

TRICEP EXTENSION – SITTING OR STANDING – BILATERAL - WEIGHT

Start with hands behind head holding free weight Extend your elbows while holding a free weight in both hands. Maintain your upper arms in an upward direction and only bend and straighten at your elbows.

	_____ Reps _____ Sets _____ X Day _____ Hold
23	**Notes:** *Neuropathy/Hands – Precaution holding weights

Starting

Position

ELBOW EXTENSION - BALL

Lie on your back on ball. Extend your elbow as shown while holding a free weight in each hand. Maintain your upper arms in an upward direction and only bend and straighten at your elbows.

	_____ Reps _____ Sets _____ X Day _____ Hold
24	**Notes:** *Neuropathy/Hands – Precaution holding weights

ELBOW EXTENSION - SKULL CRUSHER - BALL

Lie on your back on ball with a free weight in each hand. Bend your elbows to lower the weight towards the side of your head and then extend arms straight up towards the ceiling.

	_____ Reps _____ Sets _____ X Day _____ Hold
25	**Notes:**

TRICEPS - ELASTIC BAND

Fixate the band at top of door. Start with your elbow bent and holding an elastic band as shown. Pull the elastic band downward as you extend your elbow. Keep your elbow by your side the entire time.

	_____ Reps _____ Sets _____ X Day _____ Hold
26	**Notes:** *Neuropathy/Hands – Precaution holding weights

TRICEPS - BENT OVER

Stand and bend over with either support or placing your unaffected arm on thigh for support. With your targeted arm and elbow at your side, extend your elbow as you straighten your arm as shown. Keep your elbow at your side and back flat the entire time.

	_____ Reps _____ Sets _____ X Day _____ Hold
27	**Notes:**

CHAIR DIPS / PUSH UPS

While sitting in a chair with arm rests, push yourself upawards so that you lift your buttocks of the chair and then lower down controlled back to normal seated position. *If you are unable to lift yourself up, you can perform "pressure releases" so that you simply push to take some weight off your buttocks.

	_____ Reps _____ Sets _____ X Day _____ Hold
28	**Notes:**

DIPS OFF CHAIR

Push yourself up to a straight elbow position as shown. Then lower your buttocks down towards the floor by bending your elbows.

Shoulder PENDULUMS

	_____ Reps _____ Sets _____X Day _____Hold		_____ Reps _____ Sets _____X Day _____Hold
29	Notes:	**30**	Notes:

PENDULUM SHOULDER FORWARD/BACK

Shift your body weight forward then back to allow your injured arm to swing forward and back freely. Your affected arm should be fully relaxed.

PENDULUM SHOULDER – SIDE TO SIDE

Shift your body weight side to side to allow your injured arm to swing side to side freely. Your affected arm should be fully relaxed.

	_____ Reps _____ Sets _____X Day _____Hold		_____ Reps _____ Sets _____X Day _____Hold
31	Notes:	**32**	Notes: *Neuropathy/Hands – Precaution holding weights

PENDULUM SHOULDER CIRCLES
Shift your body weight in circles to allow your injured arm to swing in circles freely. Your injured arm should be fully relaxed.
REVERSE PENDULUM SHOULDER CIRCLES
Shift your body weight into reverse circles to allow your injured arm to swing in circles freely. Your injured arm should be fully relaxed.

PENDULUMS - SUPINE

Lie on your back and straighten your arm towards the ceiling. Move your arm in small circles in a clockwise motion. After a few seconds, reverse the direction to a counterclockwise motion. Change directions every few seconds.

Shoulder Flexion

_____ Reps _____ Sets _____ X Day _____ Hold	_____ Reps _____ Sets _____ X Day _____ Hold

33	Notes:	34	Notes:

ISOMETRIC FLEXION - Can use towel roll for comfort

Gently push your fist forward into a wall with your elbow bent. Hold for 5-10 seconds. Repeat.

Starting Position

SHOULDER FLEXION – SIDELYING - Can add weight

Lie on your side with arm at your side. Slowly raise the arm forward towards overhead and in front of your body.

_____ Reps _____ Sets _____ X Day _____ Hold	_____ Reps _____ Sets _____ X Day _____ Hold

35	Notes:	36	Notes: *Neuropathy/Hands – Precaution holding weights

Starting Position

FLEXION – SUPINE - SINGLE OR BILATERAL

Lie on your back with your arm at your side. Slowly raise arm up and forward towards overhead.

Starting Position

FLEXION – SUPINE – SINGLE OR BILATERAL - WEIGHT

Lie on your back with your arm at your side. Holding a weight, slowly raise arm up and forward towards overhead.

	_____ Reps _____ Sets _____X Day _____Hold

37	Notes:

Starting Position

FLEXION – SUPINE - DOWEL

Lie on your back holding dowel with both hands. Slowly raise up and forward towards overhead. Return to starting position. Repeat.
*If you have an injury/weakness, allow your unaffected arm to perform most of the effort. Your affected arm should be partially relaxed.

	_____ Reps _____ Sets _____X Day _____Hold

38	Notes:

Starting Position

FLEXION – SUPINE - DOWEL – Add weight only if equal strength

Attach ankle weight to dowel. Lie on your back holding dowel with both hands. Slowly raise up and forward towards overhead. Return to starting position. Repeat.

	_____ Reps _____ Sets _____X Day _____Hold

39	Notes:

FLEXION - SELF FIXATION – ELASTIC BAND

Hold an elastic band in front and fixate unaffected arm straight by your side or on your leg. Pull the band upward towards the ceiling with your target arm.

	_____ Reps _____ Sets _____X Day _____Hold

40	Notes:

Starting Position

FLEXION – ELASTIC BAND

In a standing position, step on the band with one leg. Keep your arm at your side holding an elastic band and draw up your arm up in front of you keeping your elbow straight.

_____ Reps _____ Sets _____ X Day _____ Hold

41 Notes:

FLEXION - STANDING - PALMS DOWN / OVERHAND DOWEL - Add weight only if equal strength

Hold a dowel/cane with both arms, palm down on both sides. Raise the dowel forward and up. (see #39/40) *Do not use weight if you have an injury/weakness. Allow your unaffected arm to perform most of the work. Your affected arm should be partially relaxed.

_____ Reps _____ Sets _____ X Day _____ Hold

42 Notes:

FLEXION - STANDING - PALMS UP /UNDERHAND DOWEL - Add weight only if equal strength

Hold a dowel/cane with both arms and palms up on both sides. Raise the dowel forward and up. *Do not use weight if you have an injury/weakness. Allow your unaffected arm to perform most of the work. Your affected arm should be partially relaxed.

_____ Reps _____ Sets _____ X Day _____ Hold

43 Notes:
*Neuropathy/Hands – Precaution holding weights

FLEXION – PALMS FACING INWARD - Can remove weight BILATERAL or ALTERNATE ARMS.

Sit or stand with your arm at your side. Hold a free weight with your palm facing your side and your elbows straight. Raise up your arm forward as shown then return to starting position. Do not let your shoulder shrug upwards unless instructed to go over shoulder level height.

_____ Reps _____ Sets _____ X Day _____ Hold

44 Notes:
*Neuropathy/Hands – Precaution holding weights

FLEXION – PALMS DOWN - Can remove weight BILATERAL or ALTERNATE ARMS.

Sit or stand with your arm at your side. Hold a weight with your palm facing down and your elbows straight. Raise up your arm forward as shown then return to starting position. Do not let your shoulder shrug upwards unless instructed to go over shoulder height.

V Raises

	_____ Reps _____ Sets _____X Day _____Hold		_____ Reps _____ Sets _____X Day _____Hold
45	Notes:	**46**	Notes: *Neuropathy/Hands – Precaution holding weights

V RAISE

Start with your arms down by your side, palms facing inward, thumbs up and your elbows straight. Raise up your arms in the form of a V to shoulder height as shown keeping elbows straight then return to starting position.

Starting Position

V RAISE – WEIGHTS

Holding free weights, start with your arms down by your side, palms facing inward and your elbows straight. Raise up your arms in the form of a V to shoulder height keeping elbows straight – return.

Shoulder Press

	_____ Reps _____ Sets _____X Day _____Hold		_____ Reps _____ Sets _____X Day _____Hold
47	Notes:	**48**	Notes: *Neuropathy/Hands – Precaution holding weights

Starting Position

MILITARY PRESS – DOWEL- Add weight only if equal strength

Hold a dowel or cane at chest height. Slowly push the wand upwards towards the ceiling until your elbows become fully straightened. Return to the original position.

Starting Position

MILITARY PRESS - FREE WEIGHTS

Hold free weights at 90-degree angle as shown above.
Slowly push your arms upwards towards the ceiling until your elbows become fully straightened. Return to the original position.

Shoulder Extension

	_____ Reps _____ Sets _____ X Day _____ Hold
49	**Notes:**

ISOMETRIC EXTENSION - Can use towel roll for comfort

Gently push your bent elbow back into a wall. Hold for 5-10 seconds. Relax and repeat.

	_____ Reps _____ Sets _____ X Day _____ Hold
50	**Notes:**

PRONE EXTENSION - EXERCISE BALL – Can add weights.

Lie face down over an exercise ball with your elbows straight and along the side of your body. Slowly raise your arms upward along your side and then return to original position.

	_____ Reps _____ Sets _____ X Day _____ Hold
51	**Notes:**

SHOULDER EXTENSION - STANDING

Start with arms by your side. Draw your arm back behind your waist. Keep your elbows straight.

	_____ Reps _____ Sets _____ X Day _____ Hold
52	**Notes:** *Neuropathy/Hands – Precaution holding weights

SHOULDER EXTENSION - STANDING - WEIGHTS

Hold a weight by your side and draw your arm back. Keep your elbows straight.

	_____ Reps _____ Sets _____X Day _____Hold
53	Notes:

Starting Position

EXTENSION – STANDING – DOWEL - Add weight only if equal strength

Hold a dowel or cane behind your back with both arms. Draw your arms back.

	_____ Reps _____ Sets _____X Day _____Hold
54	Notes:

EXTENSION - SELF FIXATION - ELASTIC BAND

Hold an elastic band out in front of you with your fixated arm. Pull the band downward towards the ground and backwards with your target arm.

	_____ Reps _____ Sets _____X Day _____Hold
55	Notes:

EXTENSION - ELASTIC BAND

Fixate the end of an elastic band at top of door. Hold the elastic band in front of you with your elbows straight. Slowly pull the band down and back towards your side.

	_____ Reps _____ Sets _____X Day _____Hold
56	Notes:

EXTENSION - BILATERAL - ELASTIC BAND

Fixate the middle of an elastic band at top of door. Hold the elastic band with both arms in front of you with your elbows straight. Slowly pull the band downwards and back towards your side.

Shoulder Internal Rotation (IR)

	_____ Reps _____ Sets _____X Day _____Hold		_____ Reps _____ Sets _____X Day _____Hold
57	Notes:	**58**	Notes:

INTERNAL ROTATION – ISOMETRIC - Can use towel roll for comfort

Press your hand into a wall using the palm side of your hand and hold. Maintain a bent elbow the entire time.

INTERNAL ROTATION - ISOMETRIC- ELEVATED - Can use towel roll for comfort

Push the front of your hand into a wall with your elbow bent and arm elevated and hold.

	_____ Reps _____ Sets _____X Day _____Hold		_____ Reps _____ Sets _____X Day _____Hold
59	Notes:	**60**	Notes:

INTERNAL ROTATION - SIDELYING

Lie on your side with your shoulder flexed to 90 degrees and elbow bent and rested on the table/bed/matt. Your forearm should be pointing up towards the ceiling. Allow your forearm to lower toward the table as shown. Place a rolled-up towel under your elbow if needed.

INTERNAL ROTATION - ELASTIC BAND

Hold an elastic band at your side with your elbow bent. Start with your hand away from your stomach and then pull the band towards your stomach. Keep your elbow near your side the entire time.

	_____ Reps _____ Sets _____X Day _____Hold
61	Notes:

	_____ Reps _____ Sets _____X Day _____Hold
62	Notes:

INTERNAL / EXTERNAL ROTATION - STANDING – DOWEL
Add weight only if equal strength

Stand and hold a dowel/cane with both hands keeping your elbows bent. Move your arms and dowel/cane side-to-side. _If you have an injury/weakness, the affected arm should be partially relaxed while your unaffected arm performs most of the effort._

Starting Position

INTERNAL ROTATION – DOWEL - Add weight only if equal strength

While holding a dowel/cane behind your back, slowly pull the wand up.

Shoulder External Rotation (ER)

	_____ Reps _____ Sets _____X Day _____Hold
63	Notes:

	_____ Reps _____ Sets _____X Day _____Hold
64	Notes:

EXTERNAL ROTATION - ISOMETRIC – Can use towel roll for comfort

Gently press your hand into a wall using the back side of your hand. Maintain a bent elbow the entire time.

EXTERNAL ROTATION - ISOMETRIC – ELEVATED - Can use towel roll for comfort

Gently push the back of your hand/arm into a wall with your arm elevated.

65	_____ Reps _____ Sets _____ X Day _____ Hold
	Notes:

Starting Position

EXTERNAL ROTATION WITH TOWEL - SIDELYING

Lie on your side with your elbow bent to 90 degrees. Place a rolled-up towel between your arm and the side your body as shown. Squeeze your shoulder blade back and rotate arm up and hold this position. Slowly rotate back to original position and repeat.

66	_____ Reps _____ Sets _____ X Day _____ Hold
	Notes: *Neuropathy/Hands – Precaution holding weights

Starting Position

EXTERNAL ROTATION – 90/90 - WEIGHTS

Hold weights with elbows bent to 90 degrees and away from your side. Rotate your shoulders back so that the palms of your hands face forward and then return as shown.

67	_____ Reps _____ Sets _____ X Day _____ Hold
	Notes:

EXTERNAL ROTATION - BILATERAL - ELASTIC BAND
Can put a towel between side and elbow (see #68)

Hold an elastic band with your elbows bent, pull your hands away from your stomach area. Keep your elbows near the side of your body.

68	_____ Reps _____ Sets _____ X Day _____ Hold
	Notes:

EXTERNAL ROTATION - ELASTIC BAND – Can add roll between side and arm

Fixate an elastic band to the door at elbow height. Hold the other end of the band at your side with your elbow bent. Start with your hand near your stomach and then pull the band away. Keep your elbow at your side the entire time.

Shoulder Adduction (ADD)

_____ Reps _____ Sets _____X Day _____Hold		_____ Reps _____ Sets _____X Day _____Hold
69	Notes:	**70**	Notes:

ADDUCTION – ISOMETRIC - Can use towel roll for comfort

Place a towel roll between your bent elbow and body. Gently push your elbow into the side of your body.

ADDUCTION - ELASTIC BAND

Fixate an elastic band to the door and hold the other end of the band away from your side. Pull the band towards your side keeping your elbow straight.

Shoulder Abduction (ABD)

_____ Reps _____ Sets _____X Day _____Hold		_____ Reps _____ Sets _____X Day _____Hold
71	Notes:	**72**	Notes:

ABDUCTION – ISOMETRIC - Can use towel roll for comfort

Gently push your elbow out to the side into a wall with your elbow bent.

HORIZONTAL ABDUCTION - DOWEL

Lie on your back holding a dowel/cane straight up towards the ceiling with your elbows straight. Bring your arms and wand to the side and then towards the other.

	_____ Reps _____ Sets _____ X Day _____ Hold
73	Notes:

HORIZONTAL ABDUCTION/ADDUCTTION - SUPINE
Lie on your back with arm straight up in front of your body.
Slowly lower your arm out towards the side. Return to
original position.

	_____ Reps _____ Sets _____ X Day _____ Hold
74	Notes: *Neuropathy/Hands – Precaution holding weights

HORIZONTAL ABDUCTION/ADDUCTTION - SUPINE -
WEIGHT

Hold a weight. Lie on your back with arm straight
up in front of your body. Slowly lower your arm
out towards the side. Return to original position

	_____ Reps _____ Sets _____ X Day _____ Hold
75	Notes:

ABDUCTION - SIDELYING - Can add weight

Lie on your side with arm at your side. Slowly raise the
target arm up towards head and away from your side.

	_____ Reps _____ Sets _____ X Day _____ Hold
76	Notes:

HORIZONTAL ABDUCTION - SIDELYING - Can add
weight

Lie on your side with arm out in front of your body.
Slowly raise up the arm overhead towards the
ceiling.

	_____ Reps _____ Sets _____X Day _____Hold
77	**Notes:** *Neuropathy/Hands – Precaution holding weights

ABDUCTION – WEIGHT – Can do without a weight

Hold a weight with your affected arm at your side. Keeping your elbow straight, raise up your arm to the side.

	_____ Reps _____ Sets _____X Day _____Hold
78	**Notes:**

ABDUCTION – ELASTIC BAND

Fixate an elastic band under a door and hold band with hand farthest away from door at your side. Keeping your elbow straight, raise up your arm to the side.

	_____ Reps _____ Sets _____X Day _____Hold
79	**Notes:**

HORIZONTAL ABDUCTION – BILATERAL - ELASTIC BAND

Hold an elastic band in both hands with your elbows straight in front of your body. Slowly pull your arms apart towards the sides.

	_____ Reps _____ Sets _____X Day _____Hold
80	**Notes:** *Neuropathy/Hands – Precaution holding weights

90/90 ABDUCTION - WEIGHT

Hold weights at your side with elbows bent to 90 degrees. Raise up your elbows away from your side while maintaining your elbows bent at 90 degrees.

Lateral/Frontal Raise

	_____ Reps _____ Sets _____X Day _____Hold		_____ Reps _____ Sets _____X Day _____Hold
81	**Notes:** *Neuropathy/Hands – Precaution holding weights	**82**	**Notes:** *Neuropathy/Hands – Precaution holding weights

Starting Position

LATERAL RAISES

Hold weights at your side with arms straight. Raise up your elbows away from your side while keeping your elbow straight the entire time.

Starting Position

LATERAL RAISES – LEAN FORWARD

Bend slightly at the waist holding weights slightly in front. Raise up your elbows away from your side squeezing shoulder blades together.

	_____ Reps _____ Sets _____X Day _____Hold		_____ Reps _____ Sets _____X Day _____Hold
83	**Notes:** *Neuropathy/Hands – Precaution holding weights	**84**	**Notes:** *Neuropathy/Hands – Precaution holding weights

Starting Position

LATERAL RAISES – LEAN FORWARD - ARM ROTATION

Bend slightly at the waist holding weights slightly in front as shown palms facing your body. Raise up your elbows away from your side squeezing shoulder blades together.

FRONTAL RAISE – WEIGHTS – Can do without weights

Hold weights at your side with arms straight. Slowly raise your arms in front of of your body.

Upright Rows

_____ Reps _____ Sets _____X Day _____Hold		_____ Reps _____ Sets _____X Day _____Hold	
85	**Notes:** *Neuropathy/Hands – Precaution holding weights	**86**	**Notes:**

Starting Position

Starting Position

UPRIGHT ROW – WEIGHTS - Can use kettle bell

Hold weights or kettlebell with both hands at waist height. Lift the weights to chest height as you bend at your elbows.

UPRIGHT ROW – ELASTIC BAND

Stand on an elastic band with either one or both feet. Hold band at waist height and raise it up to chest height as you bend at your elbows.

Shoulder Shrugs & Rolls

_____ Reps _____ Sets _____X Day _____Hold		_____ Reps _____ Sets _____X Day _____Hold	
87	**Notes:**	**88**	**Notes:** *Neuropathy/Hands – Precaution holding weights

SHRUGS

Raise your shoulders upward towards your ears as shown. Shrug both shoulders at the same time.

Starting Position

SHRUGS - WEIGHTS

Hold weights in both hands with arms straight. Raise your shoulders upward towards your ears. Shrug both shoulders at the same time.

	_____ Reps _____ Sets _____ X Day _____ Hold
89	Notes:

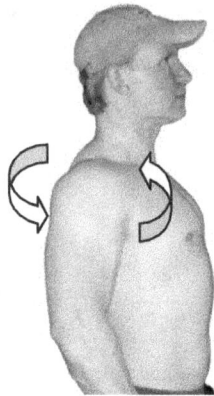

SHOULDER ROLLS

Move your shoulders in a circular pattern so that your are moving in an up, back and down direction. Perform small circles if needed for comfort.
Complete one set and then reverse direction

	_____ Reps _____ Sets _____ X Day _____ Hold
90	Notes:

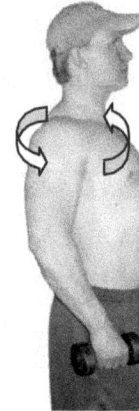

SHOULDER ROLLS - WEIGHTS

Hold weights in both or one hand. Move your shoulders in a circular pattern so that your are moving in an up, back and down direction.
Complete one set and then reverse direction

Scapular Retraction

	_____ Reps _____ Sets _____ X Day _____ Hold
91	Notes:

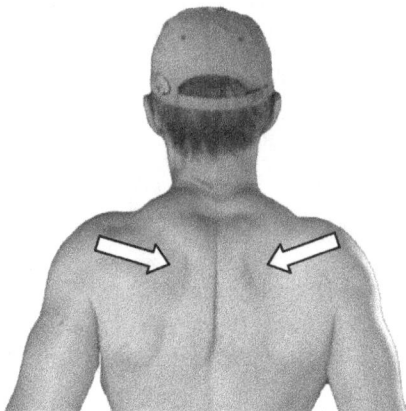

SCAPULAR RETRACTIONS - BILATERAL

Draw your shoulder blades back and down.

	_____ Reps _____ Sets _____ X Day _____ Hold
92	Notes:

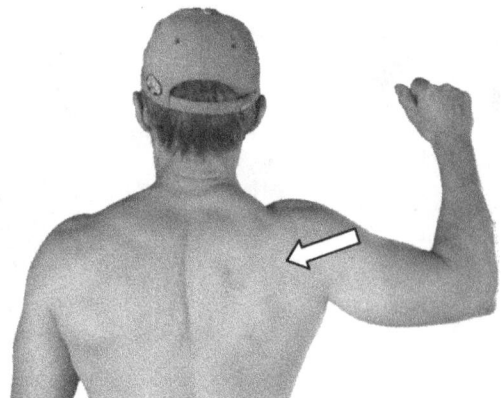

SCAPULAR RETRACTION – SINGLE ARM

With your arm raised up and elbow bent, draw your shoulder blade back and down.

	_____ Reps _____ Sets _____ X Day _____ Hold
93	**Notes:**

ELASTIC BAND SCAPULAR RETRACTIONS WITH MINI SHOULDER EXTENSIONS

Fixate an elastic band to the door and hold with both arms in front of you with your elbows straight. Slowly squeeze your shoulder blades together as you pull the band back. Be sure your shoulders do not rise up.

	_____ Reps _____ Sets _____ X Day _____ Hold
94	**Notes:** *Neuropathy/Hands – Precaution holding weights

PRONE RETRACTION – Can do without weight

Lie face down with your elbows straight. Slowly draw your shoulder blade back towards your spine. Your whole arm should rise including your shoulder blade upward as shown. Your elbow should be straight the entire time.

Scapular Protraction

	_____ Reps _____ Sets _____ X Day _____ Hold
95	**Notes:**

SCAPULAR PROTRACTION - SUPINE - BILATERAL

Lie on your back with your arms extended out in front of your body and towards the ceiling. While keeping your elbows straight, protract your shoulders reaching forward towards the ceiling. Keep your elbows straight the entire time.

	_____ Reps _____ Sets _____ X Day _____ Hold
96	**Notes:** *Neuropathy/Hands – Precaution holding weights

SCAPULAR PROTRACTION - SUPINE - WEIGHT

Lie on your back holding a weight with your arm extended out in front of your body and towards the ceiling. While keeping your elbows straight, protract your shoulders reaching forward towards the ceiling. Keep your elbows straight the entire time.

97	_____ Reps _____ Sets _____ X Day _____ Hold
	Notes:

98	_____ Reps _____ Sets _____ X Day _____ Hold
	Notes:

SCAPULAR PROTRACTION - SUPINE - ELASTIC BAND

Lie on your back and hold elastic band in both hands. Bend the unaffected arm to fixate the band. Extend the target arm out in front of your body and straight up towards the ceiling. While keeping your elbows straight, protract your shoulder blade forward towards the ceiling. Keep your elbows straight the entire time.

SCAPULAR PROTRACTION / TABLE PLANK

Start in a push up position on your hands and leaning up against a table or countertop as shown. Maintain this position as you protract your shoulder blades forward to raise your body upward a few inches. Return to original position.
*Progress by standing further away from the table.

Chest Press

99	_____ Reps _____ Sets _____ X Day _____ Hold
	Notes:

100	_____ Reps _____ Sets _____ X Day _____ Hold
	Notes: *Neuropathy/Hands – Precaution holding weights

Starting Position

CHEST PRESS – SEATED or STANDING - ELASTIC BAND

Hold elastic band with both hands at your side and elbows bent with band wrapped around body or chair. Push the band out in front of your body as you straighten your elbows.

Starting Position

CHEST PRESS – BALL, FLOOR or BENCH- WEIGHTS

Lie on your back with your elbows bent. Slowly raise up your arms towards the ceiling while extending your elbows straight up above your head.

101	_____ Reps _____ Sets _____X Day _____Hold	102	_____ Reps _____ Sets _____X Day _____Hold
	Notes:		Notes: *Neuropathy/Hands – Precaution holding weights

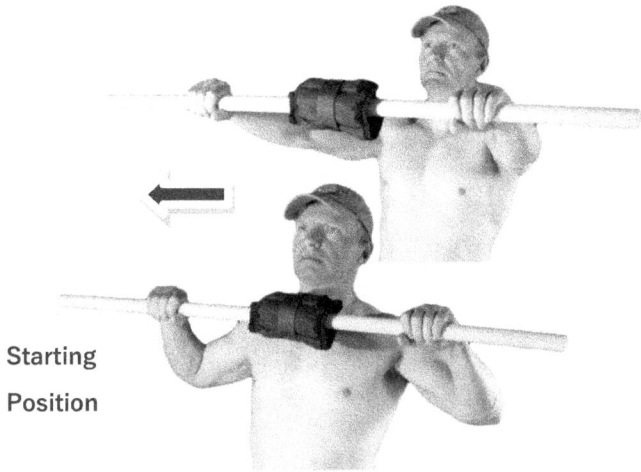

Starting
Position

DOWEL PRESS – STANDING – Add weight only if equal strength

Hold a dowel/cane at chest height. Slowly push the dowel outwards in front of your body so that your elbows become fully straightened. Return to the original position.

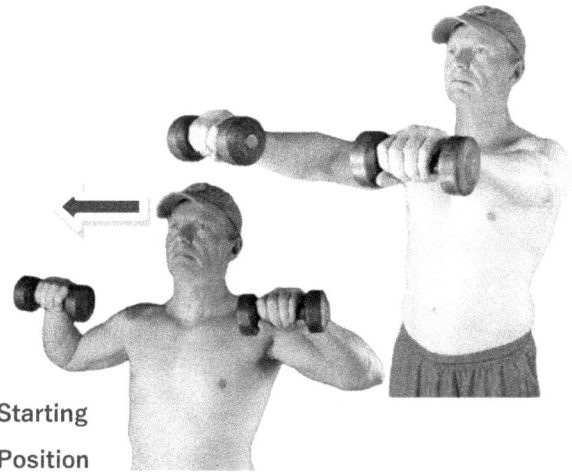

Starting
Position

CHEST PRESS – STANDING or SEATED

Hold weights in both hands with your arms at your side and elbows bent. Push your arms out in front of your body as you straighten your elbows.

Rows

103	_____ Reps _____ Sets _____X Day _____Hold	104	_____ Reps _____ Sets _____X Day _____Hold
	Notes: *Neuropathy/Hands – Precaution holding weights		Notes: *Neuropathy/Hands – Precaution holding weights

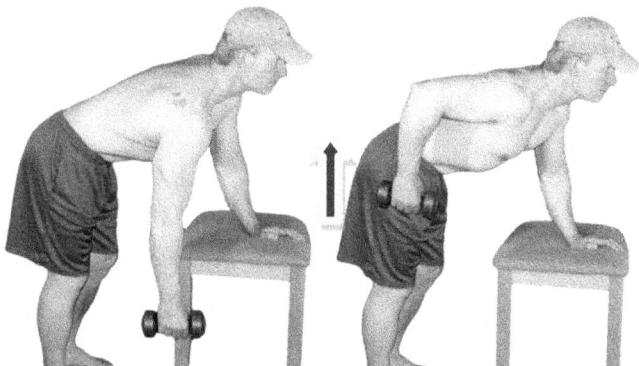

BENT OVER ROWS

Stand, bend over and support yourself with the unaffected arm. Slowly draw up your target arm as you bend your elbow. Keep your back flat the entire time.

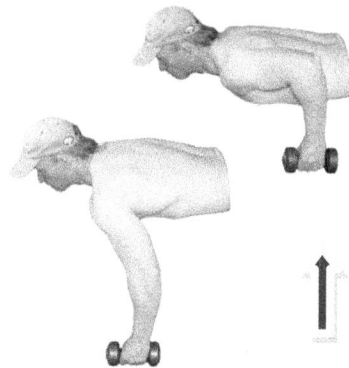

ROWS – PRONE – On bed or table

Lie face down with your elbows straight, slowly raise your arms upward while bending your elbows.

	_____ Reps _____ Sets _____X Day _____Hold
105	Notes:

ROWS - ELASTIC BAND

Fixate the elastic band in the door at elbow level. Hold the elastic band with both hands, draw back the band as you bend your elbows. Keep your elbows near the side of your body.

	_____ Reps _____ Sets _____X Day _____Hold
106	Notes:

WIDE ROWS - ELASTIC BAND

Fixate the elastic band in the door and hold the band with both hands. Draw back the band as you bend your elbows squeezing shoulder blades together. Keep your arms about 90 degrees away from the side of your body.

	_____ Reps _____ Sets _____X Day _____Hold
107	Notes:

LOW ROW – ELASTIC BAND

Fixate the elastic band in the door below elbow level. Hold the elastic band with both hands, draw back the band as you bend your elbows. Keep your elbows near the side of your body.

	_____ Reps _____ Sets _____X Day _____Hold
108	Notes:

HIGH ROW – ELASTIC BAND

Fixate the elastic band at the top of the door. Hold the elastic band with both hands, draw back the band as you bend your elbows. Keep your elbows near the side of your body.

Flys

	_____ Reps _____ Sets _____ X Day _____ Hold			_____ Reps _____ Sets _____ X Day _____ Hold
109	**Notes:** *Neuropathy/Hands – Precaution holding weights		**110**	**Notes:** *Neuropathy/Hands – Precaution holding weights

Starting

Position

FLY'S – FLOOR - WEIGHT

Holding weights, lie on your back with your arms horizontally out to the side. Bring your arms up and forward towards the ceiling. Lower your arms back down to the original position. Your elbows should be partially bent the entire time.

FLY'S – BALL or BENCH – WEIGHT

Holding weights, lie on your back on a ball with your arms horizontally out to the side. Bring your arms up and forward towards the ceiling. Lower your arms back down to the original position with elbows partially bent the entire time.

Wall pushups – To progress, move feet further away from wall

	_____ Reps _____ Sets _____ X Day _____ Hold			_____ Reps _____ Sets _____ X Day _____ Hold
111	**Notes:**		**112**	**Notes:**

WALL PUSH UPS

Place your arms out in front of you with your elbows straight so that your hands just reach the wall. Bend your elbows slowly to bring your chest closer to the wall. Straighten your arms pushing your body away from wall. Maintain your feet planted on the ground the entire time.

WALL PUSH UP - BALL

Place a ball on a wall while holding the ball with both hands as shown. Bend your elbows slowly to bring your chest closer to the wall and then straighten your arms pushing your body away from wall. Maintain your feet planted on the ground the entire time.

	_____ Reps _____ Sets _____ X Day _____ Hold
113	Notes:

WALL PUSH UP - Triceps uneven

Place your arms out in front of you with your elbows straight in an uneven position so that your hands just reach the wall. Bend your elbows slowly to bring your chest closer to the wall and then straighten your arms pushing your body away from wall. Maintain your feet planted on the ground the entire time.

	_____ Reps _____ Sets _____ X Day _____ Hold
114	Notes:

WALL PUSH UP – Hands inverted

Place your arms out in front of you with your elbows straight and hands inverted just reaching the wall. Bend your elbows slowly to bring your chest closer to the wall and then straighten your arms pushing your body away from wall. Maintain your feet planted on the ground the entire time.

	_____ Reps _____ Sets _____ X Day _____ Hold
115	Notes:

WALL PUSH UP - Narrow

Place your arms out in front of you with your elbows straight and hands close together just reaching the wall. Bend your elbows slowly to bring your chest closer to the wall and then straighten your arms pushing your body away from wall. Maintain your feet planted on the ground the entire time.

	_____ Reps _____ Sets _____ X Day _____ Hold
116	Notes:

WALL PUSH UP – Wide

Place your arms out in front of you with your elbows straight and your arms and hands far apart just reaching the wall. Bend your elbows slowly to bring your chest closer to the wall and then straighten your arms pushing your body away from wall. Maintain your feet planted on the ground the entire time.

Push ups

	_____ Reps _____ Sets _____X Day _____Hold		_____ Reps _____ Sets _____X Day _____Hold
117	Notes:	**118**	Notes:

Starting

Position

PUSH UPS - BALL

Start in a kneeling position with an exercise ball in front of you. Slowly walk yourself out with your arms so that the ball is positioned under your legs. Then perform push ups. *Progress by moving ball back towards thighs

PUSH UP - MODIFIED

Lie face down and use your arms and push yourself up. Keep your knees in contact with the floor and maintain a straight back the entire time.

	_____ Reps _____ Sets _____X Day _____Hold		_____ Reps _____ Sets _____X Day _____Hold
119	Notes:	**120**	Notes:

Starting

Position

PUSH UP

Lie face down, use your arms and push yourself. Keep your toes in contact with the floor and maintain a straight back the entire time.

PUSH UP -DIAMOND

Lie face down and place your hands on the floor in the shape of a diamond with your thumbs and index fingers.
Use your arms and push yourself up.. Keep your toes in contact with the floor and maintain a straight back the entire time.

	_____ Reps _____ Sets _____ X Day _____ Hold
121	Notes:

PUSH UP – MODIFIED - BOSU - UNSTABLE

Perform push-ups with your hands on a Bosu. Keep your knees in contact with the floor and maintain a straight back the entire time.

	_____ Reps _____ Sets _____ X Day _____ Hold
122	Notes:

PUSH UP – BOSU - UNSTABLE

Perform push-ups with your hands on top of a Bosu. Keep your toes in contact with the floor and maintain a straight back the entire time.

	_____ Reps _____ Sets _____ X Day _____ Hold
123	Notes:

PUSH UP – MODIFIED – INVERTED BOSU - UNSTABLE

Perform push-ups while holding an inverted Bosu. Try and maintain the Bosu platform as level as you can. Keep your knees in contact with the floor and maintain a straight back the entire time.

	_____ Reps _____ Sets _____ X Day _____ Hold
124	Notes:

PUSH UP – INVERTED BOSU - UNSTABLE

Perform push-ups while holding an inverted Bosu. Try and maintain the Bosu platform as level as you can. Keep your toes in contact with the floor and maintain a straight back the entire time.

BALANCE – CORE – STANDING LE STRENGTH

Basics
- Requires LE strengthening for progression
- Perform exercises 2-3x a week
- Should be performed at beginning of exercise routine or can be the main exercise routine for endurance with increased repetitions or strength with resistance.

Duration, Frequency, Intensity, Sets and Reps
- Balance – 1 set, 2-4 repetitions for hold of 5-60 seconds
- Endurance – Less than 30 second rests in between sets
  - Static - 1 set, 5-10 repetitions as tolerated
  - Dynamic – 1 set, 3-10 reps for 10-30+ second hold as tolerated
- Strengthening – Add resistance with bands or weights (*see Strengthening for more information*)
  - Static – 2-3 sets, 3-12 reps – slow controlled movements
  - Dynamic – 1-3 sets, 2-4 reps

Static Balance Progression:
1. Bilateral – Both feet on the ground
2. Unilateral – One foot on the ground
3. Arm Movement – Overhead, can do arm exercises (*See Arm Strengthening for exercises*)
4. Trunk rotation – Rotate with or without arm movement
5. Eyes Shut (lack of visual cues – sensory removal)
6. Head Turns, hand/eye tracking, shifting focal point (vestibular – sensory alteration)
7. Reading (coordination)
8. Unstable – progression
   Repeat above on unstable surface such as balance pad, pillow, balance disc or Bosu.

Decrease Base of Support (BOS) Progression:
- Wide BOS
- Narrow Bos
- Staggered/Split Stance/Semi-tandem
- Tandem Stance
- Single Leg Stance

SOLID GROUND:
1. Support: Hold onto chair, counter, sink or another stationary object.
2. No Support: Stand next to stable surface if needed for security.
   - Can start with 1-2 hands and as you become more stable, decrease the number of fingers used for support. For example, take away the thumb and hold with 4 fingers, 3 fingers, 2 fingers, 1 finger and then without support.
3. Resistance: Add ankle weights on use elastic band for resistance

UNSTABLE SURFACE: Balance pad, Bosu, Half foam roll, Pillow or Other unstable surface
1. Support: Hold onto chair, counter or another stationary object.
2. No Support: Stand next to stable surface if needed for security.
   - Can start with 1-2 hands and as you become more stable, decrease the number of fingers used for support. For example, take away the thumb and hold with 4 fingers, 3 fingers, 2 fingers, 1 finger and then without support.
3. Resistance: Add ankle weights on use elastic band for resistance

Peripheral Neuropathy **Caution Balancing on Uneven Surface**	<ul><li>Peripheral neuropathy can be a side effect of diabetes or may be as a result of damage to the peripheral nerves. These nerves carry information from the brain to other parts of the body.</li><li>Feet or lower extremity – Caution standing on uneven surface, such as a Bosu ball or balance pads due to decreased sensation in feet. Increased risk of falling.</li><li>Hands – Caution with holding dumbbells or grasping resistance bands.</li></ul>

Balance

EXERCISE Balance	EXERCISE NUMBER	NOTES
WIDE BOS DECREASING TO NARROW BOS	1	
NARROW BOS	2	
ARM MOVEMENT	3	
TRUNK ROTATION	4	
EYES SHUTS	5	
HEAD TURNS	6	
READING ALOUD	7	
BALANCE PAD	8	
SPLIT STANCE – SEMI TANDEM	9	
SPLIT STANCE - *Progression*	10	
TANDEM- SHARPENED ROMBERG STANCE	11	
TANDEM STANCE - Progression	12	
SINGLE LEG STANCE (SLS)	13	
SINGLE LEG STANCE (SLS) - *Progression*	14	
SLS – LEG FORWARD	15	
SLS – LEG BACKWARDS	16	
SLS – LEG FORWARD / OPPOSITE ARM UP	17	
SLS – LEG BACKWARDS / OPPOSITE ARM UP	18	
SLS - REACH FORWARD	19	
SLS - REACH TWIST	20	
SINGLE LEG TOE TAP	21	
SINGLE LEG STANCE - CLOCKS	22	
BALL ROLLS - HEEL TOE	23	
BALL ROLLS - LATERAL	24	
SQUAT	25	
SIT TO STAND	26	

Balance

EXERCISE	EXERCISE NUMBER	NOTES
Balance		
SQUATS – WALL WITH BALL	27	
SQUATS WITH WEIGHTS	28	
MINI SQUAT - UNSTABLE SUPPORT - FOAM PAD	29	
SQUATS - SINGLE LEG	30	
SIDE TO SIDE WEIGHT SHIFT	31	
FORWARD AND BACKWARDS WEIGHT SHIFTS	32	
SPLIT STANCE WEIGHT SHIFT SIDE TO SIDE	33	
SPLIT STANCE WEIGHT SHIFT FORWARD AND BACKWARDS	34	
WALL FALLS - FORWARD - BALANCE DRILL	35	
WALL FALLS - LATERAL - BALANCE DRILL	36	
WALL FALLS - BACKWARDS - BALANCE DRILL	37	
WALL FALLS - SINGLE LEG - FORWARD - BALANCE DRILL	38	
WALL FALLS - SINGLE LEG - LATERAL - BALANCE DRILL	39	
WALL FALLS - SINGLE LEG - MEDIAL - BALANCE DRILL	40	
WALL FALLS - SINGLE LEG - BACKWARDS - BALANCE DRILL	41	
FALL LATERAL - STEP RECOVERY	42	
FALL FORWARD - STEP RECOVERY	43	
FALL BACKWARD - STEP RECOVERY	44	
TOE TAP ABDUCTION	45	
HIP ABDUCTION - STANDING	46	
HIP EXTENSION – STANDING	47	
HIP FLEXION - STANDING – STRAIGHT LEG RAISE	48	
HIP / KNEE FLEXION - SINGLE LEG	49	
STANDING MARCHING	50	

Balance

EXERCISE	EXERCISE NUMBER	NOTES
Balance		
HAMSTRING CURL	51	
TOE RAISES	52	
TOE RAISES IR AND ER	53	
ONE LEGGED TOE RAISE	54	
SINGLE LEG BALANCE FORWARD	55	
SINGLE LEG BALANCE LATERAL	56	
SINGLE LEG BALANCE RETRO	57	
SINGLE LEG STANCE RETROLATERAL	58	
SQUAT	59	
SINGLE LEG SQUAT	60	
LUNGE – STATIC	61	
LUNGE FORWARD/BACKWARD	62	
FOUR CORNER MARCHING IN PLACE	63	
FOUR CORNER MARCHING IN PLACE WITH HEAD TURNS	64	
WALKING ON HEELS FORWARD AND BACKWARDS	65	
WALKING ON TOES FORWARD AND BACKWARDS	66	
TANDEM STANCE AND WALK – FORWARD AND BACKWARDS	67	
RUNNING MAN	68	
HOP STICK - FORWARD	69	
HOP STICK - BACKWARDS	70	
MINI LATERAL LUNGE	71	
SIDE STEPPING	72	
HOP STICK - LATERAL	73	
SINGLE LEG DEAD LIFT	74	

Balance

EXERCISE Balance	EXERCISE NUMBER	NOTES
CONE TAPS - SINGLE LEG STANCE	75	
CONE TAPS - SINGLE LEG STANCE - UNSTABLE	76	
FIGURE 8 AROUND CONES	77	
FIGURE 8 AROUND CONES – FOOT OR HAND TAP	78	
BALANCE DOUBLE LEG STANCE - WIDE	79	
BALANCE DOUBLE LEG STANCE - NARROW	80	
TANDEM STANCE	81	
TANDEM WALK	82	
SINGLE LEG STANCE - ABDUCTION	83	
SINGLE LEG STANCE - ABDUCTION	84	
SINGLE LEG STANCE – FORWARD KICK	85	
SINGLE LEG STANCE – HAMSTRING CURL	86	
SINGLE LEG SQUAT – LEG FORWARD	87	
SINGLE LEG SQUAT – LEG BACKWARDS	88	
TOE TAP OR HEEL PLACEMENT	89	
PULL UP FOOT TOUCHES ON STEP	90	
ALTERNATING SUSTAINED FOOT TOUCHES ON STEP	91	
STEP UP AND OVER	92	
FORWARD SWING THROUGH STEP	93	
SIDE STEPPING - *REPEAT STEPS 89-93 from a side approach.*	94	

BALANCE PROGRESSION- STATIC – See WARNING above Re: Peripheral Neuropathy

Hip Width/Narrow Stance >>>>> Staggered Stance >>>>> Tandem Stance   >>>>> Single-Leg Stance

1. Hold onto a chair, counter or other steady object.
2. Continue steps 2-8 holding on to a sturdy object.
3. Can start with 1-2 hands and as you become more stable, decrease the number of fingers used for support. For example, take away the thumb and hold with 4 fingers, 3 fingers, 2 fingers, 1 finger and then without support.
4. When feeling comfortable, take away support staying close to object for security
5. When able to complete with decreased support, add balance pad or unstable surface completing 2-8 as above.

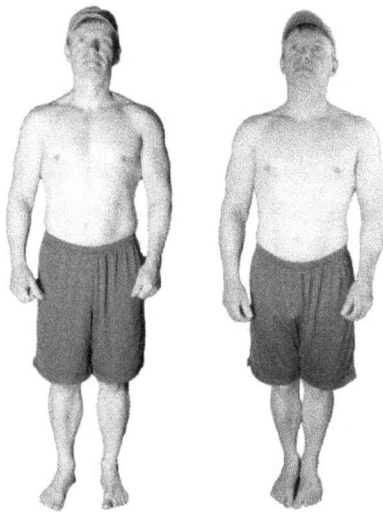

HIP WIDTH OR WIDE BASE OF SUPPORT (BOS) > NARROW BASE OF SUPPORT (BOS)

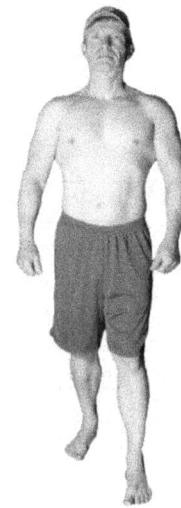

STAGGERED STANCE – SPLIT STANCE

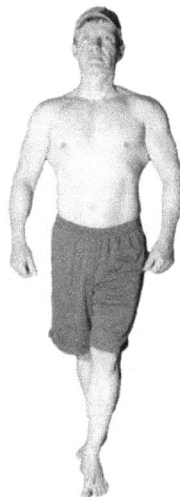

TANDEM STANCE

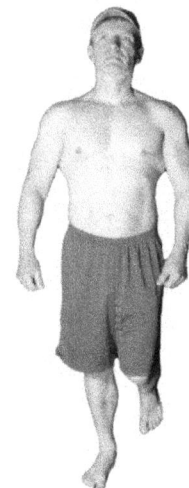

SINGLE LEG STANCE

Balance

	_____ Reps _____ Sets _____ X Day _____ Hold		_____ Reps _____ Sets _____ X Day _____ Hold
1	**Notes:**	**2**	**Notes:**

WIDE BOS DECREASING TO NARROW BOS

Continue steps 2-8 holding on to a sturdy object and then progress with decreased support as outlined above.

NARROW BOS

Stand with your feet together Count to 10. Increase time up to 60 seconds as tolerated maintaining your balance in this position.

	_____ Reps _____ Sets _____ X Day _____ Hold		_____ Reps _____ Sets _____ X Day _____ Hold
3	**Notes:**	**4**	**Notes:**

ARM MOVEMENT

Examples:
- Throw ball up in arm and catch
- Play catch with partner
- Reach hands above head and then down by side
- Do standing arm exercises (*See Arm Strengthening for examples*)

TRUNK ROTATION – reach side to side

Examples:
- Reach side to side within BOS
- Reach side to side and forward out of BOS

_____ Reps _____ Sets _____X Day _____Hold	_____ Reps _____ Sets _____X Day _____Hold

5 Notes:

6 Notes:

EYES SHUTS - Lack of visual cues – *Sensory Removal*

Stand with eyes shut and count to 10. Increase time up to 60 seconds as tolerated.

HEAD TURNS - Vestibular – *Sensory Alteration*

Examples:
- Turn head slowly from side to side
- Move head up and down slowly
- Put one finger out in front of face at arm's length moving in outward/inward direction and move head to follow with eyes. Slow hand tracking.
- Shift focal point to different objects in the room
- *Can add head turns with eyes closed*

_____ Reps _____ Sets _____X Day _____Hold	_____ Reps _____ Sets _____X Day _____Hold

7 Notes:

8 Notes:

READING ALOUD - *Coordination / Cognitive Task*

Hold reading material, such as a book, paper, tablet, or magazine in one or both hands.   Read out loud and progress to moving your head and the object on occasion to the side or up/down.

BALANCE PAD or another unstable surface

Place balance pad, Bosu, pillow or other unstable surface by a chair or counter for support. Stand on the pad.

****REPEAT STEPS 2-8 on unstable surface****

	_____ Reps _____ Sets _____ X Day _____ Hold		_____ Reps _____ Sets _____ X Day _____ Hold
9	Notes:	**10**	Notes:

SPLIT STANCE – SEMI TANDEM

Place one foot forward and the opposite foot to the back and slightly out to the side. Count to 10. Increase time up to 60 seconds as tolerated maintaining your balance in this position.

SPLIT STANCE

FOLLOW STEPS 2-8 AS SEEN WITH NARROW BOS AS OUTLINED IN BALANCE PROGRESSION

1. HOLD STEADY OBJECT PROGRESSING TO NO SUPPORT
2. STAND FOR 10-60 SECONDS
3. ARM MOVEMENT
4. TRUNK ROTATION
5. EYES SHUT
6. HEAD TURNS
7. READING
8. **UNSTABLE**

REPEAT ABOVE ON UNSTABLE SURFACE SUCH AS BALANCE PAD, PILLOW, BALANCE DISC, HALF FOARM ROLL OR BOSU.

	_____ Reps _____ Sets _____ X Day _____ Hold		_____ Reps _____ Sets _____ X Day _____ Hold
11	Notes:	**12**	Notes:

TANDEM- SHARPENED ROMBERG STANCE

Place the heel of one foot so that it touches the toes of the other foot. Count to 10. Increase time up to 60 seconds as tolerated maintaining your balance in this position.

TANDEM STANCE

FOLLOW STEPS 2-8 AS SEEN WITH NARROW BOS AS OUTLINED IN BALANCE PROGRESSION

1. HOLD STEADY OBJECT PROGRESSING TO NO SUPPORT
2. STAND FOR 10-60 SECONDS
3. ARM MOVEMENT
4. TRUNK ROTATION
5. EYES SHUT
6. HEAD TURNS
7. READING
8. **UNSTABLE**

REPEAT ABOVE ON UNSTABLE SURFACE SUCH AS BALANCE PAD, PILLOW, BALANCE DISC, HALF FOARM ROLL OR BOSU.

	_____ Reps _____ Sets _____ X Day _____ Hold		_____ Reps _____ Sets _____ X Day _____ Hold
13	Notes:	14	Notes:

SINGLE LEG STANCE (SLS)

Stand on one foot. Count to 10 > 60 seconds as tolerated maintaining your balance in this position. Maintain a slightly bent knee on the stance side.

SINGLE LEG STANCE

FOLLOW STEPS 2-8 AS SEEN WITH NARROW BOS AS OUTLINED IN BALANCE PROGRESSION

1. HOLD STEADY OBJECT PROGRESSING TO NO SUPPORT
2. STAND FOR 10-60 SECONDS
3. ARM MOVEMENT
4. TRUNK ROTATION
5. EYES SHUT
6. HEAD TURNS
7. READING
8. **UNSTABLE**

REPEAT ABOVE ON UNSTABLE SURFACE SUCH AS BALANCE PAD, PILLOW, BALANCE DISC, HALF FOARM ROLL OR BOSU.

Single Leg Stance (SLS) with Arm and/or Leg Movements- *Progress to Balance Pad*

	_____ Reps _____ Sets _____ X Day _____ Hold		_____ Reps _____ Sets _____ X Day _____ Hold
15	Notes:	16	Notes:

SLS – LEG FORWARD

Stand on one leg and maintain your balance. Hold your leg out in front of your body and then return to the original position. Repeat on opposite side. Maintain a slightly bent knee on the stance side.

SLS – LEG BACKWARDS

Stand on one leg and maintain your balance. Hold your leg in the back of your body and then return to original position. Repeat on opposite side. Maintain a slightly bent knee on the stance side.

	_____ Reps _____ Sets _____X Day _____Hold		_____ Reps _____ Sets _____X Day _____Hold
17	**Notes:**	**18**	**Notes:**

SLS – LEG FORWARD / OPPOSITE ARM UP

Stand on one leg and maintain your balance. Hold your leg out in front of your body and opposite arm up over your head. Return to the original position. Repeat on opposite side. Maintain a slightly bent knee on the stance side.

SLS – LEG BACKWARDS / OPPOSITE ARM UP

Stand on one leg and maintain your balance. Hold your leg out in front of your body and opposite arm up over your head. Return to the original position. Repeat on opposite side. Maintain a slightly bent knee on the stance side.

	_____ Reps _____ Sets _____X Day _____Hold		_____ Reps _____ Sets _____X Day _____Hold
19	**Notes:**	**20**	**Notes:**

SLS - REACH FORWARD

Stand on one leg and maintain your balance. Reach forward with your opposite arm as far as you can without losing your balance and then return to original position. Repeat on opposite side. Maintain a slightly bent knee on the stance side.

SLS - REACH TWIST

Stand on one leg and maintain your balance. Reach forward and across your body with your opposite arm as far as you can without losing your balance and then return to original position. Repeat on opposite side. Maintain a slightly bent knee on the stance side.

	_____ Reps _____ Sets _____X Day _____Hold		_____ Reps _____ Sets _____X Day _____Hold
21	Notes:	**22**	Notes:

SINGLE LEG TOE TAP

Start by standing on one leg and maintain your balance. Tap the opposite foot on a slightly raised object, such as a box or balance pad. To progress, increase the height of object, such as a stair step or cone. Can alternate feet or repeat on same side for several repetitions and then repeat on opposite side.

SINGLE LEG STANCE - CLOCKS

Start by standing on one leg and maintain your balance. Image a clock on the floor where your stance leg is in the center. Lightly touch position 1 as illustrated with the opposite foot. Then return that leg to the starting position. Next, touch position 2 and return. Maintain a slightly bent knee on the stance side.

	_____ Reps _____ Sets _____X Day _____Hold		_____ Reps _____ Sets _____X Day _____Hold
23	Notes:	**24**	Notes:

BALL ROLLS - HEEL TOE

In a standing position, place one foot on a ball and roll it forward and back in a controlled motion from heel to toe while maintaining your balance.

BALL ROLLS - LATERAL

In a standing position, place one foot on a ball and roll it side to side in a controlled motion from the inner side of your foot to the outer side of your foot while maintaining your balance.

Squats

	_____ Reps _____ Sets _____ X Day _____ Hold		_____ Reps _____ Sets _____ X Day _____ Hold
25	Notes:	**26**	Notes:

SQUAT – Can use chair or counter for support and chair behind if needed.

Stand with feet shoulder width apart (in front of a stable support for balance if needed.) Bend your knees and lower your body towards the floor. Your body weight should mostly be directed through the heels of your feet. Return to a standing position. Knees should bend in line with toes and not pass the front of the foot.

SIT TO STAND - Can use armchair to push off if needed

Start by scooting close to the front of the chair. Lean forward at your trunk and reach forward with your arms and rise to standing. (You may use a chair with arms to push off if needed and progress as tolerated).
Use your arms as a counterbalance by reaching forward when in sitting and lower them as you approach standing.

	_____ Reps _____ Sets _____ X Day _____ Hold		_____ Reps _____ Sets _____ X Day _____ Hold
27	Notes:	**28**	Notes:

SQUATS – WALL WITH BALL

Place either a small ball or therapy ball between you and the wall. Bend your knees and lower your body towards the floor. Return to a standing position. Knees should bend in line with toes and not pass the front of the foot.

SQUATS WITH WEIGHTS

Hold dumbbells or other weights in both hands by your side. Bend your knees and lower your body towards the floor. Return to a standing position. Knees should bend in line with toes and not pass the front of the foot

	_____ Reps _____ Sets _____X Day _____Hold		_____ Reps _____ Sets _____X Day _____Hold
29	Notes:	**30**	Notes:

MINI SQUAT - UNSTABLE SUPPORT - FOAM PAD

Start with your feet shoulder-width apart, toes pointed straight ahead and standing on a balance pad. Next, bend your knees to approximately 30 degrees of flexion to perform a mini squat as shown. Then, return to original position. Knees should not pass the front of the foot.

SQUATS - SINGLE LEG

While standing on one leg in front of a stable support for assisted balance, bend your knee and lower your body towards the floor. Return to a standing position.
Knees should not pass the front of the foot.

Weight Shifts, Wall Falls, Balance Recovery (Balance Drills)

	_____ Reps _____ Sets _____X Day _____Hold		_____ Reps _____ Sets _____X Day _____Hold
31	Notes:	**32**	Notes:

SIDE TO SIDE WEIGHT SHIFT
Stand next to stable surface if needed for support.

Keep feet shoulder width apart. Lean from side to side maintaining balance. *May stand in hallway with walls on both sides.*
*Advance to using balance pad

FORWARD AND BACKWARDS WEIGHT SHIFTS
Stand next to stable surface if needed for support.

Keep feet shoulder width apart. Lean from body forward and then backwards maintaining balance. *May stand in hallway with wall in front and in back.*
*Advance to using balance pad

	_____ Reps _____ Sets _____X Day _____Hold
33	**Notes:**

SPLIT STANCE WEIGHT SHIFT SIDE TO SIDE
Stand next to stable surface if needed for support.

Stand in a split stance position. Lean side to side maintaining balance. _May stand in hallway with wall on both sides._

	_____ Reps _____ Sets _____X Day _____Hold
34	**Notes:**

SPLIT STANCE WEIGHT SHIFT FORWARD AND BACKWARDS Stand next to stable surface if needed for support.

Stand in a split stance position. Lean forward and backwards maintaining balance. _May stand in hallway with wall in front and in back._

	_____ Reps _____ Sets _____X Day _____Hold
35	**Notes:**

WALL FALLS - FORWARD - BALANCE DRILL

Stand facing wall, a couple feet away from the wall. Slowly and controlled, lean forward towards the wall. Try to control your balance to prevent falling forward. Keep leaning forward gradually until eventually you do lose your balance and fall. Use your arms to catch yourself. Push yourself back upright.

	_____ Reps _____ Sets _____X Day _____Hold
36	**Notes:**

WALL FALLS - LATERAL - BALANCE DRILL

Stand to the side next to a wall, a couple feet away from the wall. Slowly and controlled, lean to the side towards the wall. Try to control your balance to prevent falling sideways. Keep leaning to the side gradually until eventually you do lose your balance and fall. Use your arm to catch yourself. Push yourself back upright.

	_____ Reps _____ Sets _____X Day _____Hold		_____ Reps _____ Sets _____X Day _____Hold
37	Notes:	38	Notes:

WALL FALLS - BACKWARDS - BALANCE DRILL

Stand facing away from a wall. Slowly and controlled, lean backward towards the wall. Try to control your balance to prevent falling backwards. Keep leaning backwards gradually until eventually you do lose your balance and fall. Use your upper back to catch the fall. Push yourself back upright.

WALL FALLS - SINGLE LEG - FORWARD - BALANCE DRILL

Stand on one leg facing a wall, a couple feet away from the wall. Slowly and controlled, lean forward towards the wall. Try to control your balance to prevent falling forward. Keep leaning forward gradually until eventually you do lose your balance and fall. Use your arms to catch yourself. Push yourself back upright.

	_____ Reps _____ Sets _____X Day _____Hold		_____ Reps _____ Sets _____X Day _____Hold
39	Notes:	40	Notes:

WALL FALLS - SINGLE LEG - LATERAL - BALANCE DRILL

Stand on one leg with a wall a couple feet off to the side of that leg. Slowly and controlled, lean to the side towards the wall. Try to control your balance to prevent falling to the side. Keep leaning gradually towards the wall until eventually you lose your balance and fall. Use your arms to catch yourself. Push yourself back upright.

WALL FALLS - SINGLE LEG - MEDIAL - BALANCE DRILL

Stand on one leg with a wall a couple feet off to the opposite side of that leg as shown. Slowly and controlled, lean sideways towards the wall. Try to control your balance to prevent falling to the side. Keep leaning gradually towards the wall until eventually you lose your balance and fall. Use your arms to catch yourself. Push yourself back upright.

	_____ Reps _____ Sets _____X Day _____Hold			_____ Reps _____ Sets _____X Day _____Hold
41	Notes:	**42**		Notes:

WALL FALLS - SINGLE LEG - BACKWARDS - BALANCE DRILL

Stand on one leg facing away from a wall. Slowly and controlled, lean backward towards the wall. Try and control your balance to prevent falling backwards. Keep leaning backwards gradually until eventually you do lose your balance and fall. Use your upper back to catch the fall. Push yourself back upright.

FALL LATERAL - STEP RECOVERY
Stand next to stable surface if needed for support.

Start in a standing position with feet apart. Slowly lean to the side and try and prevent losing your balance. Continue to lean to the side until eventually you lose your balance and need to take a step to prevent falling.

	_____ Reps _____ Sets _____X Day _____Hold			_____ Reps _____ Sets _____X Day _____Hold
43	Notes:	**44**		Notes:

FALL FORWARD - STEP RECOVERY
Stand next to stable surface if needed for support.

Start in a standing position with feet apart. Slowly lean forward and try and prevent losing your balance. Continue to lean forward until eventually you lose your balance and need to take a step to prevent falling.

FALL BACKWARD - STEP RECOVERY
Stand next to stable surface if needed for support.

Start in a standing position with feet apart. Slowly lean back and try and prevent losing your balance. Continue to lean backwards until eventually you lose your balance and need to take a step to prevent falling.

LEG EXERCISES > BALANCE > RESISTANCE

SOLID GROUND:
1. **Support:** Hold onto chair, counter, sink or another stationary object
2. **No Support:** Stand next to stable surface if needed for support
3. **Resistance:** Add ankle weights on use elastic band for resistance

UNSTABLE SURFACE: Balance pad, Bosu, Half foam roll, Pillow or Other unstable surface
1. **Support:** Hold onto chair, counter or another stationary object.
2. **No Support:** Stand next to stable surface if needed for support.
3. **Resistance:** Add ankle weights on use elastic band for resistance

Peripheral Neuropathy – See beginning of section for Caution on Unstable Surface

	_____ Reps _____ Sets _____X Day _____Hold		_____ Reps _____ Sets _____X Day _____Hold
45	Notes:	46	Notes:

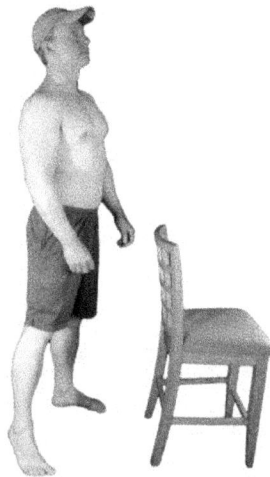

TOE TAP ABDUCTION

Standing upright and move your leg out to the side and tap your toe on the ground. Return to starting position and repeat.

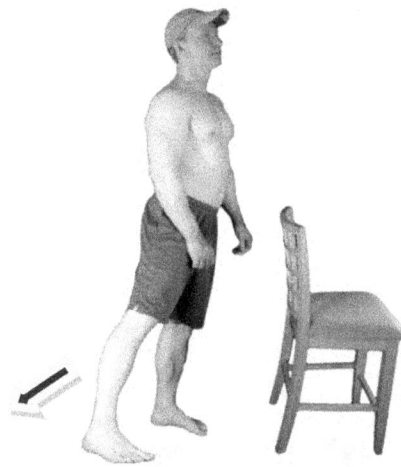

HIP ABDUCTION - STANDING – Can add ankle weights or elastic band.

Standing upright, raise your leg out to the side. Keep your knee straight and maintain your toes pointed forward the entire time. Return to starting position and repeat. Maintain a slow, controlled movement throughout.

_____ Reps _____ Sets _____X Day _____Hold		_____ Reps _____ Sets _____X Day _____Hold
47	Notes:	48

HIP EXTENSION – STANDING - Can add ankle weights or band.

Standing upright, balance on one leg and move your other leg in a backward direction. Do not swing the leg and tighten the buttock at end range. Keep your trunk stable and without arching or bending forward during the movement. Return to starting position and repeat. Maintain a slow, controlled movement throughout.

HIP FLEXION - STANDING – STRAIGHT LEG RAISE - Can add ankle weights or band.

Standing upright, balance on one leg and lift your other leg forward with a straight knee as shown. Return to starting position and repeat. Maintain a slow, controlled movement throughout.

_____ Reps _____ Sets _____X Day _____Hold		_____ Reps _____ Sets _____X Day _____Hold
49	Notes:	50

HIP / KNEE FLEXION - SINGLE LEG - Can add ankle weights

Standing upright, lift your foot and knee up, set it down. Repeat. Maintain a slow, controlled movement throughout.

STANDING MARCHING- Can add ankle weights

Standing upright, draw up your knee, set it down and then alternate to your other side. Maintain a slow, controlled movement throughout.

_____ Reps _____ Sets _____ X Day _____ Hold		_____ Reps _____ Sets _____ X Day _____ Hold
51	Notes:	**52**	Notes:

HAMSTRING CURL - Can add ankle weights.

Standing upright, balance on one leg while bending the knee of the opposite leg towards the buttocks. Return to starting position and repeat. Maintain a slow, controlled movement throughout.

TOE RAISES - Can add hand weights.

Standing upright, go up on your toes slowly towards the ceiling and then return to the starting position. Maintain a slow, controlled movement throughout.

_____ Reps _____ Sets _____ X Day _____ Hold		_____ Reps _____ Sets _____ X Day _____ Hold
53	Notes:	**54**	Notes:

TOE RAISES IR AND ER - Can add hand weights.

IR (Internal Rotation)
Standing upright, rotate feet/legs inward and go up on your toes slowly towards the ceiling and then return to the starting position. Maintain a slow, controlled movement throughout.
ER (External Rotation)
Standing upright, rotate feet/legs outward and go up on your toes slowly towards the ceiling and then return to the starting position.

ONE LEGGED TOE RAISE - Can add hand weights.

Standing upright and balance on one leg. Go up on your toes on the opposite leg towards the ceiling and then return to the starting position. Maintain a slow, controlled movement throughout.

BOSU – Can use chair for stability

	_____ Reps _____ Sets _____X Day _____Hold		_____ Reps _____ Sets _____X Day _____Hold
55	**Notes:**	**56**	**Notes:**

SINGLE LEG BALANCE FORWARD

Stand on a Bosu with one leg and maintain your balance. Hold your opposite leg out in front of your body and then return to original position. Maintain a slightly bent knee on the stance side.

SINGLE LEG BALANCE LATERAL

Stand on a Bosu with one leg and maintain your balance. Hold your opposite leg out to the side of your body and then return to original position. Maintain a slightly bent knee on the stance side.

	_____ Reps _____ Sets _____X Day _____Hold		_____ Reps _____ Sets _____X Day _____Hold
57	**Notes:**	**58**	**Notes:**

SINGLE LEG BALANCE RETRO

Stand on a Bosu Ball with one leg and maintain your balance. Hold your opposite leg back behind your body and then return to original position. Maintain a slightly bent knee on the stance side.

SINGLE LEG STANCE RETROLATERAL

Stand on a Bosu Ball with one leg and maintain your balance. Hold your opposite leg back behind and across your body and then return to original position. Maintain a slightly bent knee on the stance side.

	_____ Reps _____ Sets _____X Day _____Hold
59	Notes:

SQUAT

While standing and maintaining your balance on a Bosu, squat and return to a standing position. Knees should bend in line with the 2nd toe and not pass the front of the foot.

	_____ Reps _____ Sets _____X Day _____Hold
60	Notes:

SINGLE LEG SQUAT

While standing and balancing on a Bosu with one leg, bend your knee and lower your body towards the ground. Return to a standing position. Your stance knee should bend in line with the 2nd toe and not pass the front of the foot.

Lunges

	_____ Reps _____ Sets _____X Day _____Hold
61	Notes:

Starting Position

LUNGE – STATIC

Start in standing position with back leg straight and front leg with flexed/bent knee. Lean forward on front knee keeping knee in line with foot and back leg remaining straight. Return to starting position and repeat for several repetitions and then repeat on opposite side.
*Make sure front knee does not go past the foot.

	_____ Reps _____ Sets _____X Day _____Hold
62	Notes:

Backward   Starting Position   Forward

LUNGE FORWARD/BACKWARD

Start in standing (*middle picture*).
Backward: Keep one foot planted and step back with the opposite foot. Return to original position - repeat. *Forward:* Keep one foot planted and step forward with the opposite foot. Return to original position - repeat.

DYNAMIC MOVEMENTS

	_____ Reps _____ Sets _____X Day _____Hold
63	**Notes:**

FOUR CORNER MARCHING IN PLACE

Marching in place, move your body clockwise stopping at each corner for several seconds and move to the next corner. After completing the square, march counterclockwise.

	_____ Reps _____ Sets _____X Day _____Hold
64	**Notes:**

FOUR CORNER MARCHING IN PLACE WITH HEAD TURNS

With Head and Body Moving Simultaneously
March in place to four corners, as previous exercise (#63). Move your head and body moving simultaneously as you complete the square.
With Head Turn And Then Body Turn.
March in place to four corners, as previous exercise (#63). Turn head and then body as you complete the square.

	_____ Reps _____ Sets _____X Day _____Hold
65	**Notes:**

WALKING ON HEELS FORWARD AND BACKWARDS – May walk along kitchen counter or wall until feeling steady.

Standing up tall, walk forward on heels. After feeling secure with a forward motion, try walking backwards on heels.

	_____ Reps _____ Sets _____X Day _____Hold
66	**Notes:**

WALKING ON TOES FORWARD AND BACKWARDS – May walk along kitchen counter or wall until feeling steady.

Standing up tall, walk forward on up on toes. After feeling secure with a forward motion, try walking backwards up on toes.

_____ Reps _____ Sets _____ X Day _____ Hold

67 Notes:

TANDEM STANCE AND WALK – FORWARD AND
BACKWARDS

Maintaining your balance, stand with one foot directly in
front of the other so that the toes of one foot touches the
heel of the other. Progress by taking steps with your heel
touching your toes with each step.
**Progress by walking backwards with your toe touching
your heel with each step. Can also add head turns.

_____ Reps _____ Sets _____ X Day _____ Hold

68 Notes:

RUNNING MAN

Stand and balance on one leg. Lean forward as you
bring your other leg back behind you to tap the
floor. Bring the same side arm forward as shown
during the movement. Return to starting position
and repeat.

_____ Reps _____ Sets _____ X Day _____ Hold

69 Notes:

HOP STICK - FORWARD

Stand on one leg and then hop forward onto the other
leg. Maintain your balance the entire time. Increase the
difficulty by hoping forward further or higher.

_____ Reps _____ Sets _____ X Day _____ Hold

70 Notes:

HOP STICK - BACKWARDS

Stand on one leg and then hop backward onto the
other leg. Maintain your balance the entire time.
Increase the difficulty by hoping back further or
higher.

	_____ Reps _____ Sets _____X Day _____Hold
71	Notes:

MINI LATERAL LUNGE

Step to the side and balance on the leg. Next return to the original position. Repeat in the opposite direction. Your knees should be bent about 30 degrees.

	_____ Reps _____ Sets _____X Day _____Hold
72	Notes:

SIDE STEPPING – May step along kitchen counter or in hallway for support.

Step to the side continuing for length of room or counter – repeat in opposite direction.

	_____ Reps _____ Sets _____X Day _____Hold
73	Notes:

HOP STICK - LATERAL

Stand on one leg and then hop to the side onto the other leg. Maintain your balance the entire time. Increase the difficulty by hoping to the side further and higher.

	_____ Reps _____ Sets _____X Day _____Hold
74	Notes:

SINGLE LEG DEAD LIFT

While standing on one leg, bend forward with arms in front towards the ground as you extend your leg behind you and then return to the original position. Keep your legs straight and maintain your balance the entire time.

	_____ Reps _____ Sets _____X Day _____Hold		_____ Reps _____ Sets _____X Day _____Hold
75	Notes:	**76**	Notes:

CONE TAPS - SINGLE LEG STANCE

Place 3-5 cones or cups around you as shown. Balance on a slightly bent knee. Lower yourself down to tap the top of a cone with your finger. Return to original position and repeat touching a different cone. Advance exercise with smaller cones/cups and or faster speed.

CONE TAPS - SINGLE LEG STANCE - UNSTABLE

Place 3-5 cones or cups around you. Balance on an unstable surface such as a foam pad with a slightly bent knee. Lower yourself down to tap the top of a cone. Return to original position and repeat touching a different cone. Advance exercise with smaller cones/cups and or faster speed.

	_____ Reps _____ Sets _____X Day _____Hold		_____ Reps _____ Sets _____X Day _____Hold
77	Notes:	**78**	Notes:

FIGURE 8 AROUND CONES

Set up 4-8 cones on the floor about 12 inches apart, although can vary to increase or decrease difficulty. Weave in and out of cones and then turn and repeat.

FIGURE 8 AROUND CONES – FOOT OR HAND TAP

Follow #75 figure around 4- 8 cones. To increase difficulty, you can tap each cone with your foot or lean over and tap with your hand.

HALF ROLLER (static and dynamic) – FLAT SIDE UP OR DOWN

_____ Reps _____ Sets _____X Day _____Hold		_____ Reps _____ Sets _____X Day _____Hold

79	Notes:	80	Notes:

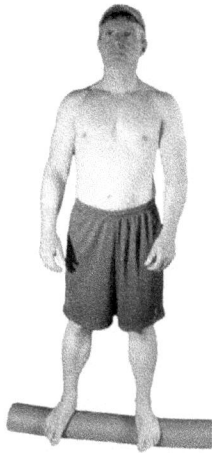

BALANCE DOUBLE LEG STANCE - WIDE

Place a half foam roll on the ground in a side-to-side direction. Stand on the foam roll with your feet spread apart and maintain your balance.

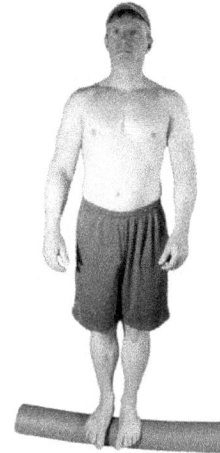

BALANCE DOUBLE LEG STANCE - NARROW

Place a half foam roll on the ground in a side-to-side direction. Stand on the foam roll with your feet together and maintain your balance.

_____ Reps _____ Sets _____X Day _____Hold		_____ Reps _____ Sets _____X Day _____Hold

81	Notes:	82	Notes:

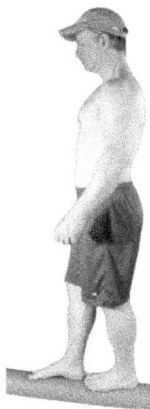

TANDEM STANCE

Place a half foam roll on the ground in a forward-back direction. Stand on the foam roll in tandem stance (with your heel and toe touching as shown) and maintain your balance.

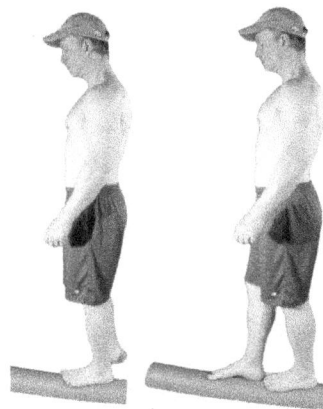

TANDEM WALK

Place a half foam roll on the ground in a forward-back direction. Stand on the foam roll and begin tandem walking (heel-toe pattern walking as shown). Once you get to the end of the roll, either turn around or tandem walk backward.

	_____ Reps _____ Sets _____X Day _____Hold		_____ Reps _____ Sets _____X Day _____Hold
83	**Notes:**	**84**	**Notes:**

SINGLE LEG STANCE - ABDUCTION

Place a half foam roll on the ground in a side-to-side direction. Balance on one leg and move the opposite leg to the side.

SINGLE LEG STANCE - ABDUCTION

Place a half foam roll on the ground in a forward-back direction. Balance on one leg with the opposite leg to the side.

	_____ Reps _____ Sets _____X Day _____Hold		_____ Reps _____ Sets _____X Day _____Hold
85	**Notes:**	**86**	**Notes:**

SINGLE LEG STANCE – FORWARD KICK

Place a half foam roll on the ground in a forward-back direction. Balance on one leg and move the opposite leg forward.

SINGLE LEG STANCE – HAMSTRING CURL

Place a half foam roll on the ground in a forward-back direction. Balance on one leg and with the opposite leg, bend the knee backwards as shown.

	_____ Reps _____ Sets _____ X Day _____ Hold
87	Notes:

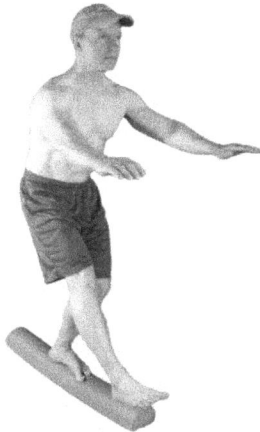

SINGLE LEG SQUAT – LEG FORWARD

Place a half foam roll on the ground in a forward-back direction. Balance on one leg with a slight bend in the supporting knee and move the opposite leg forward. Straighten supporting knee and repeat.

	_____ Reps _____ Sets _____ X Day _____ Hold
88	Notes:

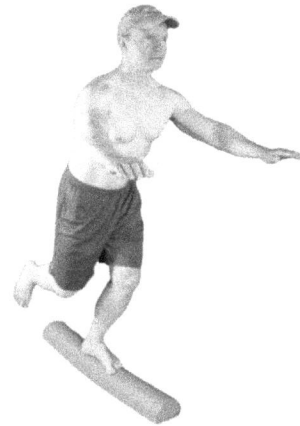

SINGLE LEG SQUAT – LEG BACKWARDS

Place a half foam roll on the ground in a forward-back direction. Balance on one leg with a slight bend in the supporting knee and with the opposite leg, move the leg backwards as shown with bent knee. Straighten supporting knee and repeat.

STAIR STEP – *To progress, increase step height*

	_____ Reps _____ Sets _____ X Day _____ Hold
89	Notes:

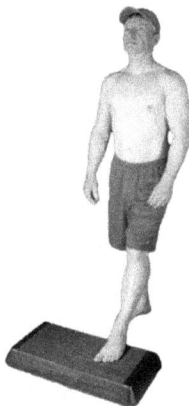

TOE TAP OR HEEL PLACEMENT

While standing with both feet on the floor, place one foot on the top of the step. Next, return the foot back to the floor and then repeat with the other leg.
You can either put your foot up for several repetitions or alternate.

	_____ Reps _____ Sets _____ X Day _____ Hold
90	Notes:

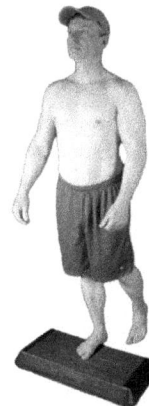

PULL UP FOOT TOUCHES ON STEP

Whie standing with both feet on the ground, put one foot on the step. Push through the foot straightening the knee until the opposite foot is off the ground. Lower the foot back to the starting position. Repeat with the opposite foot for several repetitions.

	_____ Reps _____ Sets _____ X Day _____ Hold
91	Notes:

ALTERNATING SUSTAINED FOOT TOUCHES ON STEP

Whie standing with both feet on the ground, put one foot on the step. Push through the foot straightening the knee until the opposite foot is also on the step. Step off backwards to the starting position. Repeat with the opposite foot for several repetitions.

	_____ Reps _____ Sets _____ X Day _____ Hold
92	Notes:

STEP UP AND OVER

Step up onto the step and then onto the ground on the other side. Turn around and repeat.
Repeat several repetitions on one side and then the other or alternate legs.

	_____ Reps _____ Sets _____ X Day _____ Hold
93	Notes:

FORWARD SWING THROUGH STEP

Step up onto the step without stopping on the top, swing opposite leg through and onto the floor on the other side.

	_____ Reps _____ Sets _____ X Day _____ Hold
94	Notes:

SIDE STEPPING

******REPEAT STEPS 89-93 from a side approach******

Agility

EXERCISE Agility/Reactivity/Speed	EXERCISE NUMBER	NOTES
Four Square Drills	1	
Dots	2	
Ladder Drills	3	
Box Drills	4	
Cones	5	
Hurdles	6	

Agility/Reactivity/Speed

According to the Twist Conditioning workbook, "Agility is the ability to link several fundamental movement skills into a multidirectional pattern. Reaction skills are the 'whole body' responsiveness to external stimuli, as well as muscle and joint internal reactivity. Quickness is the ability to explosively initiate movement from a stationary position, as well as shifting the gears of speed". (*Twist, Peter, Twist Agility, Quickness and & Reactivity Workbook, 2009, pg 16*)

Agility is a combination of acceleration, deceleration, coordination, power, strength and dynamic balance. With agility training, always keep your head in a neutral position looking straight ahead no matter which way you turn. "Powerful arm movement during transitional and directional changes is essential in order to reacquire a high rate of speed". (*Brown & Ferrigno, 2005, pp 73-74*)

Agility exercises can be done with cones, hurdles, dots or squares on the floor, box drills, Bosu or ladders. Agility can also be high impact or explosive movements. If you are not comfortable with this in the beginning or have any contraindications, stick with low impact movements. In other words, if you are jumping over hurdles, keep them low to the ground and jump over with one leg leading for low impact and jump with both legs for high impact.

If you are doing box drills or Bosu, please do NOT JUMP off backwards.

AGILITY / SPEED / REACTIVITY

4 Square Drills

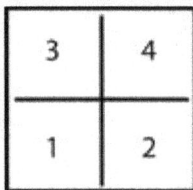 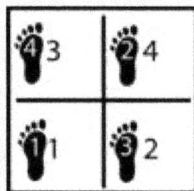 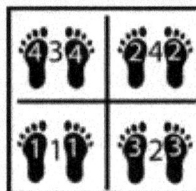 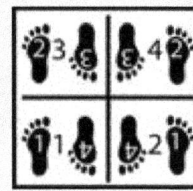

Dots

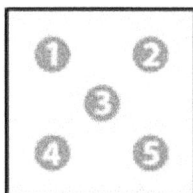 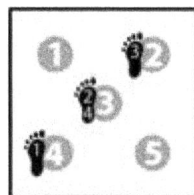 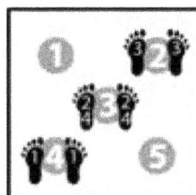 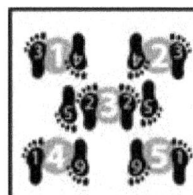

Ladder

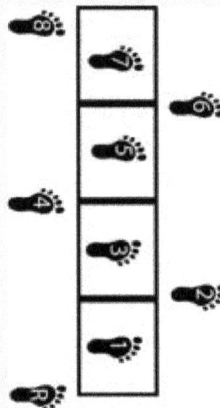 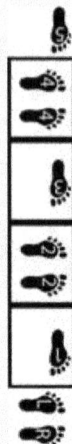 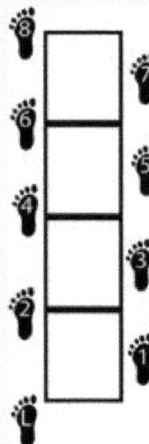 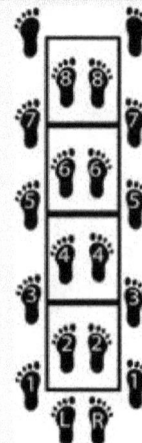

Box Drills – Box should be no higher than the middle of your shin. This can be done on Bosu for balance.

Alt Tap Box With Foot	Down Up Both Feet Together	Quickly Move Side to Side	Down Up Both Feet Together
Switch			

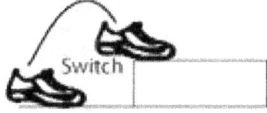

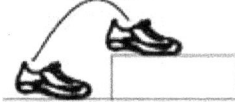

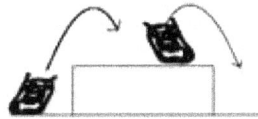

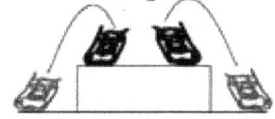

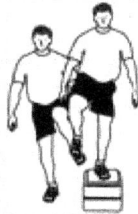

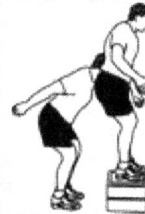

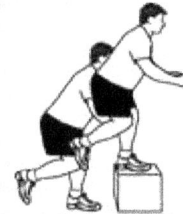

Cones

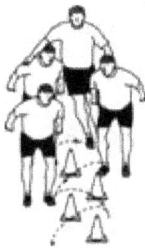

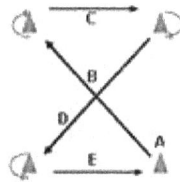

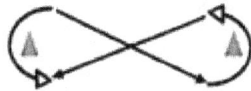

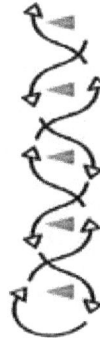

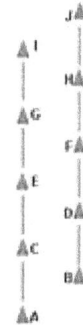

Hurdles – can run or jump over hurdles

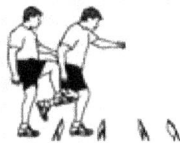

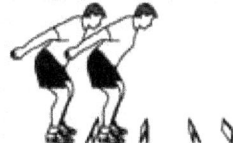

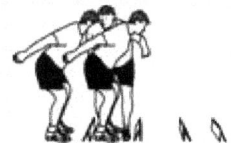

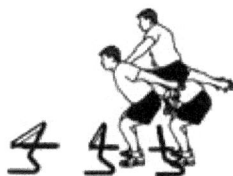

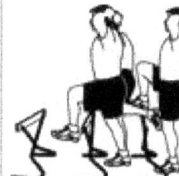

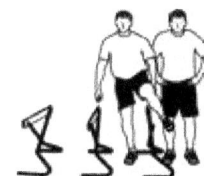

Endurance / Aerobic Capacity

Aerobic - with oxygen: Muscular and Cardiovascular

Many repetitions with sub-maximal weight (weight that is less than the maximum you can lift).

Muscular endurance is the ability of the muscle or group of muscles to sustain repeated contractions against resistance for an extended period of time. This is needed to build muscle. (See *Strengthening*). Cardiovascular endurance is the ability of the heart, lungs and blood vessels to deliver oxygen to working muscles and tissues, as well as the ability of those muscles and tissues to utilize that oxygen. This is needed to help endure long runs or sustained activity, as with biking or running. In short, endurance or aerobic exercises increase the heart rate and respiratory rate.

As far as long-term performance goes, there are two types of muscle fibers that can determine the likelihood of success: slow and fast twitch, which may determine whether you are more likely to be a power-lifter or sprinter (*fast twitch*), or a marathon runner (*slow twitch*). Your ability depends on the distribution of these fibers in the body. In other words, you could have a certain percentage of slow twitch in your biceps, but a different percentage in your quadriceps. There is some controversy over whether you can change the percentage or distribution of these fibers with endurance training or training for a specific event, although you may be able to change the glycolytic capacity.

Type of Fibers	***Slow twitch fibers:*** Have a high aerobic capacity and are resistant to fatigue. People that have a higher percentage of slow twitch fibers tend to have better endurance abilities. ***Fast twitch fibers:*** Contract faster than slow twitch, and thus fatigue faster. People that have a higher percentage of fast twitch fibers tend to have better sprinting or muscle building abilities.

The following research is from the: **MAYO CLINIC**

Mayo Clinic - *https://www.mayoclinic.org/healthy-lifestyle/fitness/in-depth/aerobic-exercise/art-20045541*

Regular aerobic activity, such as walking, bicycling or swimming, can help you live longer and healthier. Need motivation? See how aerobic exercise affects your heart, lungs and blood flow.

How your body responds to aerobic exercise

During aerobic activity, you repeatedly move large muscles in your arms, legs and hips. You'll notice your body's responses quickly.

You'll breathe faster and more deeply. This maximizes the amount of oxygen in your blood. Your heart will beat faster, which increases blood flow to your muscles and back to your lungs.

Your small blood vessels (capillaries) will widen to deliver more oxygen to your muscles and carry away waste products, such as carbon dioxide and lactic acid.

Your body will even release endorphins, natural painkillers that promote an increased sense of well-being.

What aerobic exercise does for your health.

Regardless of age, weight or athletic ability, aerobic activity is good for you. As your body adapts to regular aerobic exercise, you will get stronger and fitter.

Consider the following 10 ways that aerobic activity can help you feel better and enjoy life to the fullest on the next page.

Aerobic activity can help you:

1. **Keep excess pounds at bay**
   Combined with a healthy diet, aerobic exercise helps you lose weight and keep it off.

2. **Increase your stamina**
   You may feel tired when you first start regular aerobic exercise. But over the long term, you'll enjoy increased stamina and reduced fatigue.

3. **Ward off viral illnesses**
   Aerobic exercise activates your immune system in a good way. This may leave you less susceptible to minor viral illnesses, such as colds and flu.

4. **Reduce your health risks**
   Aerobic exercise reduces the risk of many conditions, including obesity, heart disease, high blood pressure, type 2 diabetes, metabolic syndrome, stroke and certain types of cancer.

   Weight-bearing aerobic exercises, such as walking, help decrease the risk of osteoporosis.

5. **Manage chronic conditions**
   Aerobic exercise may help lower blood pressure and control blood sugar. If you have coronary artery disease, aerobic exercise may help you manage your condition.

6. **Strengthen your heart**
   A stronger heart doesn't need to beat as fast. A stronger heart also pumps blood more efficiently, which improves blood flow to all parts of your body.

7. **Keep your arteries clear**
   Aerobic exercise boosts your high-density lipoprotein (HDL), the "good," cholesterol, and lowers your low-density lipoprotein (LDL), the "bad," cholesterol. This may result in less buildup of plaques in your arteries.

8. **Boost your mood**
   Aerobic exercise may ease the gloominess of depression, reduce the tension associated with anxiety and promote relaxation.

9. **Stay active and independent as you age**
   Aerobic exercise keeps your muscles strong, which can help you maintain mobility as you get older. Studies have found that regular physical activity may help protect memory, reasoning, judgment and thinking skills (cognitive function) in older adults and may improve cognitive function in young adults.

10. **Live longer**
    Studies show that people who participate in regular aerobic exercise live longer than those who don't exercise regularly.

Take the first step

Ready to get more active? Great. Just remember to start with small steps. If you've been inactive for a long time or if you have a chronic health condition, get your doctor's OK before you start. When you're ready to begin exercising, start slowly. You might walk five minutes in the morning and five minutes in the evening.
The next day, add a few minutes to each walking session. Pick up the pace a bit, too. Soon, you could be walking briskly for at least 30 minutes a day and reaping all the benefits of regular aerobic activity.

Other options for aerobic exercise could include cross-country skiing, aerobic dancing, swimming, stair climbing, bicycling, jogging, elliptical training or rowing.

(Mayo Clinic - *https://www.mayoclinic.org/healthy-lifestyle/fitness/in-depth/aerobic-exercise/art-20045541*)

Calories

Calorie: A unit of food energy. The word calorie is ordinarily used instead of the more precise, scientific term kilocalorie. A kilocalorie represents the amount of energy required to raise the temperature of a liter of water 1' centigrade at sea level. Technically, a kilocalorie represents 1,000 true calories of energy. *(MedicineNet.com)*

Calories are a measurement tool, like inches or cups. Calories measure the energy a food or beverage provides from the carbohydrate, fat, protein, and alcohol* it contains. Calories give you the fuel or energy you need to work and play – even to rest and sleep! When choosing what to eat and drink, it's important to get the right mix – enough nutrients without too many calories. Paying attention to calories is an important part of managing your weight. The amount of calories you need are different if you want to gain, lose, or maintain your weight. Tracking what and how much you eat, and drink can help you better understand your calorie intake over time. Each person's body may have different needs for calories and exercise. A healthy lifestyle requires balance in the foods you eat, the beverages you drink, the way you do daily activities, adequate sleep, stress management, and in the amount of activity in your daily routine. *(ChooseMyPlate.gov & CDC)*

Example of Activities and Calories Burned (*ChooseMyPlate.gov*)
A 154-pound man who is 5' 10" will use up (burn) about the number of calories listed doing each activity below. Those who weigh more will use more calories; those who weigh less will use fewer calories. The calorie values listed include both calories used by the activity and the calories used for normal body functioning during the activity time.

EXAMPLE	Approximate calories used (burned) by a 154-pound man	
MODERATE physical activities:	In 1 hour	In 30 minutes
Hiking	370	185
Light gardening/ yard work	330	165
Dancing	330	165
Golf (walking and carrying clubs)	330	165
Bicycling (less than 10 mph)	290	145
Walking (3.5 mph)	280	140
Weight training (general light workout)	220	110
Stretching	180	90
VIGOROUS physical activities:	In 1 hour	In 30 minutes
Running/ jogging (5 mph)	590	295
Bicycling (more than 10 mph)	590	295
Swimming (slow freestyle laps)	510	255
Aerobics	480	240
Walking (4.5 mph)	460	230
Heavy yard work (chopping wood)	440	220
Weightlifting (vigorous effort)	440	220
Basketball (vigorous)	440	220

References

Also, Some Good Books, Websites & DVD'

ACE Idea Fitness Journal*: Martina M. Cartwright, PhD, RD http://www.ideafit.com/fitness-library/protein-today-are-consumers-getting-too-much-of-a-good-thing?ACE_ACCESS=ebec6bcf61abff08f7b1d8b27c555758*

ACE Senior Fitness Manual, *American Council on Exercise* (2014)

American Physical Therapy Association, (APTA), 2007. *Basic Science for Animal Physical Therapy: Canine, 2nd edition*

Arleigh J Reynolds, DVM, PhD - *www.absasleddogracing.org.uk/newgang/src/gangline/role.htm*

Australian Institute of Sports - *http://www.ausport.gov.au*

BodyBuilder.com

Brown & Ferrigno, (2005). *Training for Speed, Agility and Quickness*, Champaign, IL: Human Kinetics.

Bryant, C & Green, D, editors (2003), *Ace Personal Trainer Manual, 3rd ed.*, San Diego, CA: American Council on Exercise (ACE)

ChooseMyPlate.gov

Examine.com

ExRx.net

Feher & Szunyoghy (1996). *Cyclopedia Anatomicae,* Tess Press

Gillette, R (2002). Temperature Regulation of the Dog. Retrieved June 2011 from *http://www.sportsvet.com/11Nwsltr.PDF*

Gillette, R (2008). *Feeding the Canine Athlete for Optimal Performance.* Retrieved September 25, 2008 from *www.sports vet.com/Art3.html.*

Glucose (Wikipedia) - *http://en.wikipedia.org/wiki/Glucose*

Glycemic Index (Wikipedia) - *http://en.wikipedia.org/wiki/Glycemic_index*

LiveStrong.com

Mayo Clinic - *https://www.mayoclinic.org/healthy-lifestyle/fitness/in-depth/aerobic-exercise/art-20045541*

MedicineNet.com

Myofascial Release: (Wikipedia) - https://en.wikipedia.org/wiki/Myofascial_release

Rikli, Roberta and Jones, Jessie (2013) *Senior Fitness Test Manual, 2nd Ed.,*

Strength Training: (Wikipedia) *http://en.wikipedia.org/wiki/Strength_training*

Twist, Peter (2009). *Twist Agility, Quickness and & Reactivity Workbook.* British Columbia: Twist Conditioning, Inc. University of Maryland Medical Center.com

Workout Australia

Thank You to:

My Husband
Model

For his support through my battle with cancer and while writing this and previous books.
Also, for the patience and hours he put in modeling for this book.

My Daughter

For giving me artistic inspiration and providing artwork for my previous books.

My Grandchildren
Just Because

God

For giving me the strength to overcome cancer and the wisdom to write these books.

Certifications, Continuing Education and License

Physical Therapist Assistant – L/PTA – 30 years in both Home Therapy and Short-Term Rehab facilities

ACE Certified Personal Trainer – CPT
- o **Functional Training Specialist**
- o **Therapeutic Exercise Specialist**
- o **Senior Fitness Specialist**
- o **Nutrition and Fitness Specialist**

©Klose Education
- o **Certified Lymphedema Therapist – CLT**
- o **Strength After Breast Cancer – Strength ABC**
- o **Breast Cancer Rehabilitation**

©Cancer Exercise Specialist Institute – CETI
- o **Cancer Exercise Specialist – CES**
- o **Breast Cancer Recovery BOSU(R) Specialist Advanced Qualification**
- o **Pilates Mat Certificate**

©MedFit
- o **Medical Fitness Specialist**
- o **Parkinson's Disease Fitness Specialist**
- o **Arthritis Fitness Specialist**

©Pink Ribbon Program

©The BioMechanics Method - Corrective Exercise Specialist

©ISSA - DNA-Based Fitness Coach

www.ingramcontent.com/pod-product-compliance
Lightning Source LLC
Chambersburg PA
CBHW052110020426
42335CB00021B/2705